Malaria Control and Elimination in China

Xiao-Nong Zhou • Jian-Hai Yin
Editors

Malaria Control and Elimination in China

Case Studies

Springer

Editors
Xiao-Nong Zhou
National Institute of Parasitic Diseases at Chinese Center for Disease Control and Prevention (Chinese Center for Tropical Diseases Research); National Key Laboratory of Intelligent Tracking and Forecasting for Infectious Diseases; NHC Key Laboratory of Parasite and Vector Biology; WHO Collaborating Centre for Tropical Diseases; National Center for International Research on Tropical Diseases, Ministry of Science and Technology
Shanghai, People's Republic of China

School of Global Health, Chinese Center for Tropical Diseases Research, Shanghai Jiao Tong University School of Medicine
Shanghai, People's Republic of China

Hainan Center for Tropical Diseases Research (Sub-Center of the Chinese Center for Tropical Diseases)
Haikou, People's Republic of China

Jian-Hai Yin
School of Global Health, Chinese Center for Tropical Diseases Research, Shanghai Jiao Tong University School of Medicine
Shanghai, People's Republic of China

ISBN 978-981-97-8718-0 ISBN 978-981-97-8719-7 (eBook)
https://doi.org/10.1007/978-981-97-8719-7

This Springer imprint is published by the registered company Springer Nature Singapore Pte Ltd.
The registered company address is: 152 Beach Road, #21-01/04 Gateway East, Singapore 189721, Singapore

Preface

Malaria, the most fatal mosquito-borne illness globally, holds a distinct place as one of the "Big Three" infectious diseases, alongside HIV/AIDS and tuberculosis. Despite the increasing number of countries achieving pre-elimination or malaria elimination status, the disease remains a significant threat to human life and health worldwide. In 2022, an estimated 249 million malaria cases and 608,000 malaria-related deaths recorded in 85 malaria-endemic countries. Remarkably, over 90% of these malaria cases and 95% of malaria-related fatalities occurred in Africa.

The diligent documentation of national triumphs in eradicating malaria is pivotal in demonstrating the efficacy of this crucial public health endeavor. It is also essential for disseminating valuable insights from established practices and encouraging greater political backing from governments. China, following seven decades of relentless efforts in malaria control and elimination, received malaria-free certification from the World Health Organization on June 30, 2021. The garnered knowledge can benefit other malaria-stricken countries in advancing their respective elimination programs. From China's malaria control and elimination programs, five crucial lessons emerge: First, a consistent political commitment, coupled with adequate organizational and financial support, along with technical expertise, is imperative for the thorough implementation of national malaria control and elimination strategies. Second, scientifically tailored response strategies and measures, tailored to the varying settings and stages, produced cost-effective outcomes. Third, the national malaria elimination program relies heavily on practical multisectoral collaborations, including social mobilization, community engagement, and effective cross-border partnerships. Fourth, robust and effective interventions, such as standardized management, rigorous quality control of techniques, and timely responses to malaria outbreaks, are crucial for achieving the malaria-free status, supported by web-based reporting systems and a robust network of malaria diagnostic reference laboratories. Finally, unwavering scientific and technological innovation in control and elimination strategies, pathogen detection methods, and the development of new antimalarial drugs accelerates the eradication process in China.

In the ongoing post-elimination phase, our unwavering dedication remains focused on preventing the re-establishment of malaria transmission stemming from imported cases and mitigating malaria-related fatalities. Simultaneously, China has been proactively aligning itself with the malaria elimination goal outlined in the United Nations' Sustainable Development Goals, standing ready to collaborate with nations worldwide under the tutelage and coordination of the World Health Organization. To further promote cross-country and cross-regional cooperation, initiatives have been devised to foster information sharing and experience exchange, thereby broadening the avenues to contribute China's insights to the global malaria elimination program. While the journey to malaria elimination differs among countries, the cornerstones of success remain universally applicable. Recently, a panel of over 30 experts, led by Professor Xiao-Nong Zhou and Dr. Jian-Hai Yin from the National Institute of Parasitic Diseases at the Chinese Center for Disease Control and Prevention (Chinese Center for Triopical Diseases Research), reviewed and documented China's pivotal learnings in the malaria control and elimination quest. These insights, supported by the Bill and Melinda Gates Foundation (Grant No. INV-018913), can serve as valuable reference points for malaria-endemic countries. Here, we extend our profound gratitude to the esteemed members of the advisory committee, including Dr. Ning Xiao and Dr. Zhi-Gui Xia of the National Institute of Parasitic Diseases at the Chinese Center for Disease Control and Prevention (Chinese Center for Triopical Diseases Research), Dr. Xiao-Peng Qi and Dr. Li-Jie Zhang from the Chinese Center for Disease Control and Prevention, Prof. Jeanette Rainey of the US Centers for Disease Control and Prevention, as well as Dr. Xiao-Yu Wei and Prof. Fu-Jie Xu from the Bill and Melinda Gates Foundation. Their invaluable perspectives and recommendations have significantly enriched the quality of each chapter.

In this book, *Malaria Control and Elimination in China*: *Case Studies*, seven diverse case studies from various subregions of China, encompassing distinct epidemiological and socioeconomic landscapes, are presented. These encompass (1) a case-based malaria surveillance and response, highlighting the implementation of the 1-3-7 approach in Jiangsu Province; (2) a study on malaria along the international border in Yunnan, China, spanning 2003–2020, focusing on border malaria control and elimination; (3) the utilization of a layer strategy (LS) to promote malaria elimination among Hainan's forest dwellers; (4) insights on ensuring the efficacy of mass drug administration in controlling *Plasmodium vivax* malaria; (5) the role of bacterial larvicides in containing malaria outbreaks; and (6) two case studies tracing the discovery history and international promotion of artemisinin.

China has indeed intensified its technical cooperation and pilot projects in malaria control and elimination, collaborating with various countries affected by malaria. Specifically, it has fostered and enhanced joint malaria prevention and control mechanisms with numerous countries in the Lancang-Mekong region at the borders, taking decisive measures to jointly tackle the threat of antimalarial drug resistance in the region. Another China–Australia–Papua New Guinea Malaria Control Pilot Project has been underway since 2016. In Africa, the China–UK–Tanzania Malaria Control Pilot Project in Tanzania has been successfully implemented since 2015, with public health cooperation, including malaria control and elimination, being a key priority in the China–Africa Cooperation Forum and the Belt and Road Initiative.

It is anticipated that the experiences shared from China's malaria control and elimination programs in this publication will aid in progressing from malaria control to elimination, thereby bolstering the global malaria elimination program, namely the E-2025 initiative.

Shanghai, People's Republic of China Xiao-Nong Zhou
Shanghai, People's Republic of China Jian-Hai Yin

Contents

Editors and Contributors

About the Editors

Xiao-Nong Zhou National Institute of Parasitic Diseases at Chinese Center for Disease Control and Prevention (Chinese Center for Tropical Diseases Research); National Key Laboratory of Intelligent Tracking and Forecasting for Infectious Diseases; NHC Key Laboratory of Parasite and Vector Biology; WHO Collaborating Centre for Tropical Diseases; National Center for International Research on Tropical Diseases, Ministry of Science and Technology; School of Global Health, Chinese Center for Tropical Diseases Research, Shanghai Jiao Tong University School of Medicine, Shanghai, PR China; Hainan Center for Tropical Diseases Research (Sub-Center of the Chinese Center for Tropical Diseases), Haikou, PR China.

Jian-Hai Yin National Institute of Parasitic Diseases at Chinese Center for Disease Control and Prevention (Chinese Center for Tropical Diseases Research); National Key Laboratory of Intelligent Tracking and Forecasting for Infectious Diseases; NHC Key Laboratory of Parasite and Vector Biology; WHO Collaborating Centre for Tropical Diseases; National Center for International Research on Tropical Diseases, Ministry of Science and Technology; Shanghai, PR China.

Contributors

Jun Cao Key Laboratory of National Health Commission (NHC) on Parasitic Disease Control and Prevention, Jiangsu Provincial Key Laboratory on Parasite and Vector Control Technology, Jiangsu Institute of Parasitic Diseases, Wuxi, Jiangsu, People's Republic of China

School of Public Health, Center for Global Health, Nanjing Medical University, Nanjing, Jiangsu, People's Republic of China

Yuan-Yuan Cao Key Laboratory of National Health Commission (NHC) on Parasitic Disease Control and Prevention, Jiangsu Provincial Key Laboratory on Parasite and Vector Control Technology, Jiangsu Institute of Parasitic Diseases, Wuxi, Jiangsu, People's Republic of China

Qi-Yan Chen Yunnan Institute of Parasitic Diseases, Puer, Yunnan, People's Republic of China

Yan Deng Henan Center for Disease Control and Prevention, Zhengzhou, Henan, People's Republic of China

Zhi-Quan He Henan Center for Disease Control and Prevention, Zhengzhou, Henan, People's Republic of China

Xiao-Min Huang Hainan Provincial Center for Disease Control and Prevention, Haikou, Hainan, People's Republic of China

Yang-Mu Huang Department of Global Health, Peking University School of Public Health, Peking University, Beijing, People's Republic of China

Institute for Global Health, Peking University, Beijing, People's Republic of China

Jing-Jing Jiang Anhui Provincial Center for Disease Control and Prevention, Hefei, Anhui, People's Republic of China

Wei-Dong Li Anhui Provincial Center for Disease Control and Prevention, Hefei, Anhui, People's Republic of China

Yu-Chun Li Hainan Provincial Center for Disease Control and Prevention, Haikou, Hainan, People's Republic of China

Guang-Qi Liu Department of Global Health, Peking University School of Public Health, Peking University, Beijing, People's Republic of China

Institute for Global Health, Peking University, Beijing, People's Republic of China

Hui Liu Yunnan Institute of Parasitic Diseases, Puer, Yunnan, People's Republic of China

Ying Liu Henan Center for Disease Control and Prevention, Zhengzhou, Henan, People's Republic of China

Yu-Ming Liu Department of Global Health, Peking University School of Public Health, Peking University, Beijing, People's Republic of China

Institute for Global Health, Peking University, Beijing, People's Republic of China

Xiao-Feng Lv Anhui Provincial Center for Disease Control and Prevention, Hefei, Anhui, People's Republic of China

Feng Meng Hainan Provincial Center for Disease Control and Prevention, Haikou, Hainan, People's Republic of China

Dan Qian Henan Center for Disease Control and Prevention, Zhengzhou, Henan, People's Republic of China

Ding-Wei Sun Hainan Provincial Center for Disease Control and Prevention, Haikou, Hainan, People's Republic of China

Yi-Nuo Sun Department of Global Health, Peking University School of Public Health, Peking University, Beijing, People's Republic of China

Institute for Global Health, Peking University, Beijing, People's Republic of China

Dan Wang Hainan Provincial Center for Disease Control and Prevention, Haikou, Hainan, People's Republic of China

Henan Center for Disease Control and Prevention, Zhengzhou, Henan, People's Republic of China

Guang-Ze Wang Hainan Provincial Center for Disease Control and Prevention, Haikou, Hainan, People's Republic of China

Jian-Jun Wang Anhui Provincial Center for Disease Control and Prevention, Hefei, Anhui, People's Republic of China

Shuai Wang Hainan Provincial Center for Disease Control and Prevention, Haikou, Hainan, People's Republic of China

Shu-Qi Wang Anhui Provincial Center for Disease Control and Prevention, Hefei, Anhui, People's Republic of China

Wei-Ming Wang Key Laboratory of National Health Commission (NHC) on Parasitic Disease Control and Prevention, Jiangsu Provincial Key Laboratory on Parasite and Vector Control Technology, Jiangsu Institute of Parasitic Diseases, Wuxi, Jiangsu, People's Republic of China

Yan Xie Department of Global Health, Peking University School of Public Health, Peking University, Beijing, People's Republic of China

Institute for Global Health, Peking University, Beijing, People's Republic of China

Jian-Wei Xu Yunnan Institute of Parasitic Diseases, Puer, Yunnan, People's Republic of China

Xian Xu Anhui Provincial Center for Disease Control and Prevention, Hefei, Anhui, People's Republic of China

Jian-Hai Yin School of Global Health, Chinese Center for Tropical Diseases Research, Shanghai Jiao Tong University School of Medicine, Shanghai, People's Republic of China

Wen Zeng Hainan Provincial Center for Disease Control and Prevention, Haikou, Hainan, People's Republic of China

Cang-Lin Zhang Yunnan Institute of Parasitic Diseases, Puer, Yunnan, People's Republic of China

Tao Zhang Anhui Provincial Center for Disease Control and Prevention, Hefei, Anhui, People's Republic of China

Hua-Yun Zhou Key Laboratory of National Health Commission (NHC) on Parasitic Disease Control and Prevention, Jiangsu Provincial Key Laboratory on Parasite and Vector Control Technology, Jiangsu Institute of Parasitic Diseases, Wuxi, Jiangsu, People's Republic of China

Xiao-Nong Zhou National Institute of Parasitic Diseases, at Chinese Center for Disease Control and Prevention (Chinese Center for Tropical Diseases Research); National Key Laboratory of Intelligent Tracking and Forecasting for Infectious Diseases; NHC Key Laboratory of Parasite and Vector Biology; WHO Collaborating Centre for Tropical Diseases; National Center for International Research on Tropical Diseases, Ministry of Science and Technology, Shanghai, People's Republic of China

School of Global Health, Chinese Center for Tropical Diseases Research, Shanghai Jiao Tong University School of Medicine, Shanghai, People's Republic of China

Hainan Center for Tropical Diseases Research (Sub-Center of the Chinese Center for Tropical Diseases), Haikou, People's Republic of China

Yao-Wu Zhou Yunnan Institute of Parasitic Diseases, Yunnan Provincial Centre of Malaria Research, Puer, Yunnan, People's Republic of China

Guo-Ding Zhu Key Laboratory of National Health Commission (NHC) on Parasitic Disease Control and Prevention, Jiangsu Provincial Key Laboratory on Parasite and Vector Control Technology, Jiangsu Institute of Parasitic Diseases, Wuxi, Jiangsu, People's Republic of China

Center for Global Health, School of Public Health, Nanjing Medical University, Nanjing, Jiangsu, People's Republic of China

Chapter 1
Case Study on Malaria Surveillance and Response: Implementation of the 1-3-7 Approach in Jiangsu Province, China

Yuan-Yuan Cao, Hua-Yun Zhou, Wei-Ming Wang, Guo-Ding Zhu, and Jun Cao

Learning Objectives

Upon completion of this case study, participants should be able to

1. Comprehend the background and significance of the 1-3-7 approach.
2. Identify the key measures and prerequisites of the 1-3-7 approach.
3. Understand the implementation of malaria elimination in Jiangsu Province.
4. Discuss the challenges and strategies in executing the 1-3-7 approach.

Since the initiation of China's National Malaria Elimination Action Plan (NMEAP) in 2010, the 1-3-7 surveillance and response apporach have been devised and implemented nationwide to support the malaria elimination program. The 1-3-7 approach has significantly contributed to the achievement of the elimination objectives. As of 2017, China has successfully halted indigenous malaria transmission. This case study focuses on the way of implementation of the 1-3-7 approach during malaria elimination program in Jiangsu Province as a notable example.

Y.-Y. Cao · H.-Y. Zhou · W.-M. Wang
Key Laboratory of National Health Commission (NHC) on Parasitic Disease Control and Prevention, Jiangsu Provincial Key Laboratory on Parasite and Vector Control Technology, Jiangsu Institute of Parasitic Diseases, Wuxi, Jiangsu, People's Republic of China

G.-D. Zhu (✉) · J. Cao (✉)
Key Laboratory of National Health Commission (NHC) on Parasitic Disease Control and Prevention, Jiangsu Provincial Key Laboratory on Parasite and Vector Control Technology, Jiangsu Institute of Parasitic Diseases, Wuxi, Jiangsu, People's Republic of China

School of Public Health, Center for Global Health, Nanjing Medical University, Nanjing, Jiangsu, People's Republic of China

X.-N. Zhou, J.-H. Yin (eds.), *Malaria Control and Elimination in China*,
https://doi.org/10.1007/978-981-97-8719-7_1

1.1 Part 1. Overview of Surveillance and Response in Malaria Elimination

In 2015, the World Health Organization (WHO) introduced the Global Technical Strategy for Malaria 2016–2030 (GTS) (WHO 2015) (Fig. 1.1), outlining the vision and objectives for a malaria-free world. The shared vision among WHO and countries at risk of malaria is a global elimination of the disease. Specific targets have been set for 2020, 2025, and 2030, including reducing global malaria mortality rates and case incidence compared to 2015.

China achieved WHO certification as malaria-free in June 2021, becoming the first country in the WHO Western Pacific Region to receive such recognition in over three decades. After a 70-year endeavor, China's successful malaria elimination efforts led to this prestigious certification, marking a remarkable milestone for a country that once reported 30 million annual malaria cases in the 1940s.

Surveillance and response (S&R) have been identified as key interventions for malaria elimination (Fig. 1.2). The GTS outlines three pillars and two supporting elements (e.g., Pillar 1, Pillar 2, and Pillar 3) crucial for this endeavor (WHO 2017). Transforming malaria surveillance into a core intervention under Pillar 3 of the GTS represents a strategic shift necessary as the focus transitions from control to elimination.

Question and Answer

1. How to implement the three pillars in Global Technical Strategy in your country?

Reference answers 1:

– It is an open question and there is no standard answer.

Proposed discussion time:

– 3 min.

Vision: A world free of malaria

Goals	Milestones		Targets
	2020	2025	2030
1. Reduce malaria mortality rates globally compared with 2015	≥40%	≥75%	≥90%
2. Reduce malaria case incidence globally compared with 2015	≥40%	≥75%	≥90%
3. Eliminate malaria from countries in which malaria was transmitted in 2015	At least 10 countries	At least 20 countries	At least 35 countries
4. Prevent re-establishment of malaria in all countries that are malaria-free	Re-establishment prevented	Re-establishment prevented	Re-establishment prevented

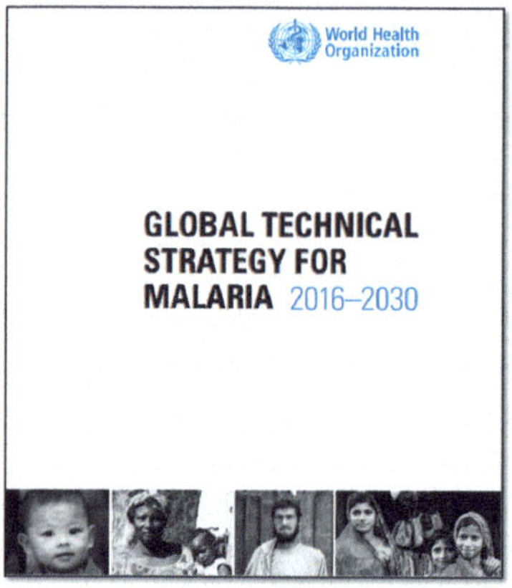

Global **Malaria** Programme World Health Organization 3

Fig. 1.1 Global Technical Strategy for Malaria 2016–2030 (GTS)

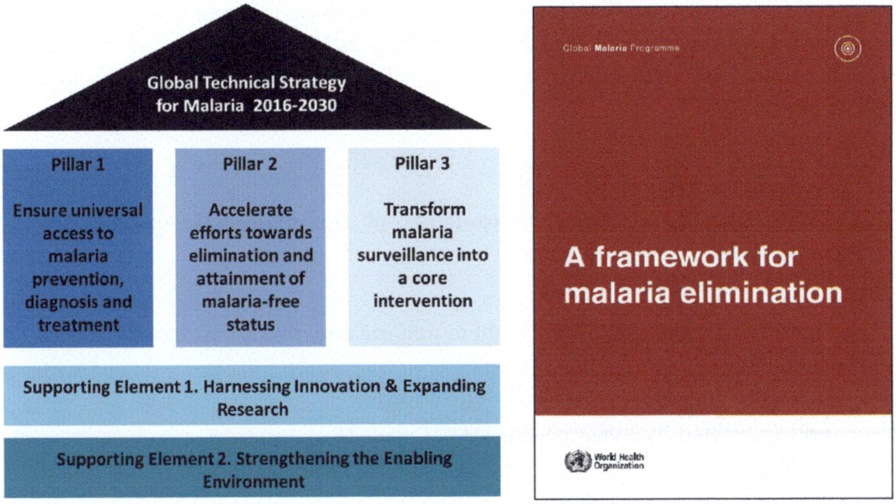
Global Technical Strategy for Malaria 2016-2030
Pillar 1
Ensure universal access to malaria prevention, diagnosis and treatment
Pillar 2
Accelerate efforts towards elimination and attainment of malaria-free status
Pillar 3
Transform malaria surveillance into a core intervention
Supporting Element 1. Harnessing Innovation & Expanding Research
Supporting Element 2. Strengthening the Enabling Environment
Global Malaria Programme
A framework for malaria elimination
World Health Organization

Fig. 1.2 Global Technical Strategy 2016–2030 and a framework for malaria elimination issued by the World Health Organization

1.2 Part 2. Background of the 1-3-7 Malaria Surveillance Response Approach

1.2.1 Malaria Epidemic Trends in China and Globally

Malaria remains one of the most significant infectious diseases that poses a serious threat to global health and security. In 2019, there were still 215 million reported cases of malaria, resulting in approximately 384 thousand deaths, with the majority of cases concentrated in sub-Saharan Africa, Southeast Asia, and Latin America (WHO 2020). In China, the 1940s saw over 30 million annual malaria infections, severely compromising public health and impeding social and economic progress (Tang 1999). The 1960s and 1970s witnessed two major malaria outbreaks, respectively. Through substantial government involvement and effective leadership, malaria control efforts have yielded significant results over the past decades. By 2009, nationwide malaria cases had decreased to 14,000, reported from 87 counties across 24 malaria-endemic provinces (Zhou et al. 2011). Building on this progress in the control phase, China initiated the National Malaria Elimination Action Plan (NMEAP) in 2010, aiming to achieve elimination by 2020. Since the launch of NMEAP, the endemic malaria burden has seen a drastic reduction. In 2017, local malaria transmission was successfully interrupted for the first time nationwide in China (Feng et al. 2018), leading to China's official certification as malaria-free by the WHO in June 2021.

Jiangsu Province was among the highly endemic regions for malaria in China, with an annual incidence rate peaking at 24.95% in the 1960s. Through a comprehensive approach involving control of mosquito-borne transmission sources, standardized treatment for malaria cases, and mass drug administration (MDA), Jiangsu Province managed to reduce the annual malaria incidence to 0.1 per 10,000 for three consecutive years from 2008 to 2010. The local malaria cases in Jiangsu Province plummeted from over 1000 in 2001 to just 13 in 2011 (Zhou et al. 2013). Aligned with the NMEAP, Jiangsu Province launched its provincial malaria elimination action plan in 2010.

Question and Answer

2. What are the primary components of the diagnostic criteria for malaria cases?

Reference answers 2:

- Epidemiological history: traveled to malaria endemic areas, blood transfusion history.
- Clinical symptoms: fever, chilling, sweating.
- Lab examination: microscopy, RDT (Fig. 1.3).

Proposed discussion time:

- 5 min.

Travelers visiting malaria-endemic regions and spending nights in areas with malaria transmission are at higher risk of malaria infection. Symptoms such as chilling, fever, and sweating are commonly experienced by malaria patients during the onset of the disease. Ultimately, malaria diagnosis relies on one of several examinations, including microscopy, rapid diagnosis tests (RDTs), and polymerase chain reaction (PCR) tests.

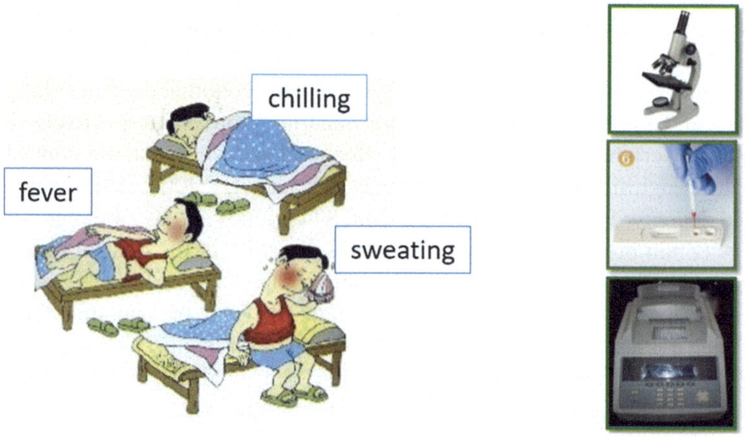

Fig. 1.3 Major components of diagnostic criteria for malaria cases

1.2.2 Transition from Control to Elimination in China

In China, the transition from the control phase to the elimination phase has brought about significant changes in the characteristics of the malaria epidemic. During the control phase, the focus was on population-based interventions. However, in the malaria elimination phase, China has shifted its strategy toward case-based sensitive surveillance and rapid response.

There are six key differences between the control phase and the elimination phase in terms of surveillance and response approaches (Table 1.1). The crucial shift involves moving from "targeting high-incidence areas and reducing the incidence" with a focus on population prevention and control to "targeting each outbreak with case intervention at the core." To effectively interrupt malaria transmission in broader regions, three determinations must be reinforced during this transition for timely interruption of malaria transmission, including (1) timely detection of the infection source, (2) identification of the infection source, and (3) pinpointing the location of infection (Lei and Wang 2012).

1.2.3 Timely Seeking Health-Care Services

The effectiveness of malaria elimination program can be hindered by two types of time delays: patient delay and medical diagnostic delay, as indicated in a systematic review (Fig. 1.4) (Bastaki et al. 2018). Firstly, patient delay, also known as delay in seeking health care (PD), refers to the period between the onset of symptoms and the first visit to a medical facility or health-care provider. Patient delays in seeking health care contribute significantly to the overall diagnostic delay. Secondly, medical treatment delay (MTD) is defined as the time from the initial medical consultation or seeking health-care advice to the commencement of malaria treatment. Therefore, timely healthcare-seeking by malaria patients plays a crucial role in the early detection of malaria cases.

Table 1.1 Differences in control and elimination phases

Items	Control stage	Elimination stage
Goal and strategy	Reduce morbidity and mortality	Block local transmissions
Work mode	Population-based	Case-based
Target	High endemic areas/population	Focus/foci with malaria transmission risk
Population	All susceptible people in endemic areas	People who may be infected through malaria cases and surrounding
Intervention	Population-based (MDA, ITN, and IRS)	Individual case based (each case and foci)
Indicator	Coverage	Timeline

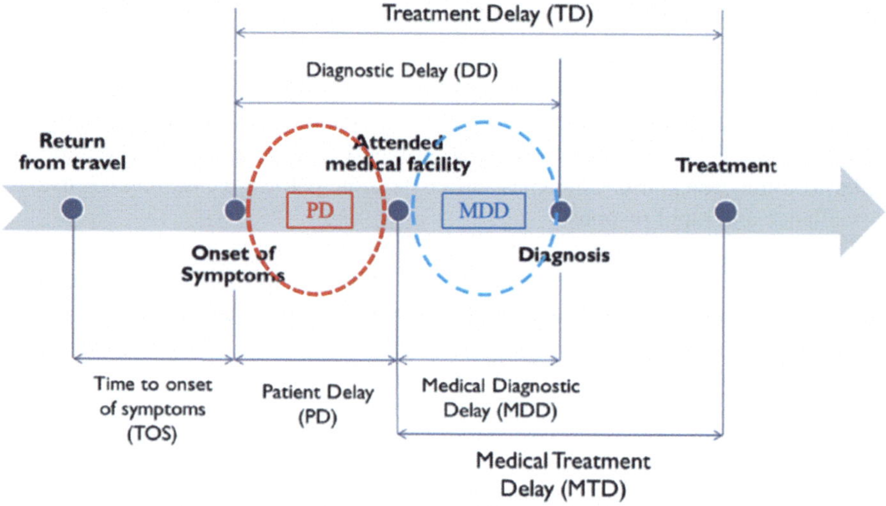

Fig. 1.4 Major delays for malaria diagnosis. (From *Travel Med Infect Dis* 2018)

Question and Answer

3. How can the prompt seeking of health-care services for malaria patients be enhanced?

Reference answers 3:

- It remains an open question.

Proposed discussion time:

- 5 min

4. How can the timeliness and accuracy of malaria diagnosis be improved?

Reference answers 4:

- This question is open-ended, and there is no definitive answer.

Proposed discussion time:

- 5 min

1.2.4 China's 1-3-7 Surveillance and Response Approach

In response to the challenges and critical issues confronting the national malaria elimination program and the imperative to achieve the goal of malaria elimination, we are actively exploring innovative approaches in surveillance and response systems (Cao et al. 2013) (Table 1.1), with a specific emphasis on promptly interrupting malaria transmission. Taking into account the dynamics of malaria transmission, we have introduced the "1-3-7" surveillance and response approach for malaria elimination, which highlights three key measures, their respective stakeholders, and time frames. This approach outlines a series of coordinated actions to be executed within specific time frames, as depicted in Fig. 1.5.

Within 1 day: Any instance of malaria must be reported within 24 h through China's routine disease surveillance information system (CRDSIS). All health-care facilities are mandated to report malaria cases, including suspected ones, directly via the web-based CRDSIS within 1 day (24 h).

Within 3 days: Each malaria case must undergo scrutiny and epidemiological investigation completed within 3 days. Health professionals from the county-level centers for disease control and prevention (CDCs) in the area where the malaria case is reported are responsible for verifying cases through laboratory tests and confirmations within this time frame. Simultaneously, these professionals need to conduct on-site epidemiological investigations to identify the *Plasmodium* species and trace the sources of infection.

Within 7 days: The malaria focus must be identified and addressed within a week. Health professionals from the county-level CDCs in the region where the malaria case is located are tasked with determining the risk of transmission through focus investigations within 7 days. Concurrently, these CDCs must implement targeted measures to manage the malaria focus based on investigation findings. Epidemiological surveys will focus on assessing the identification of malaria

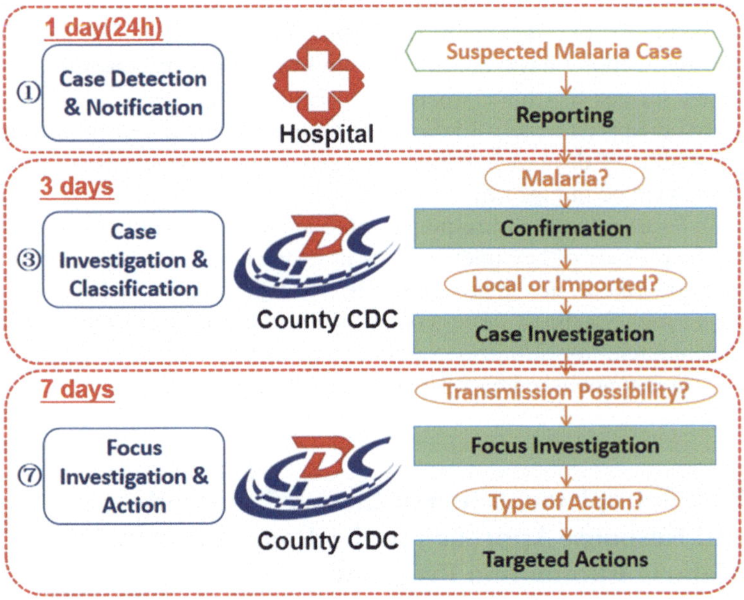

Fig. 1.5 Schematic time windows for the chain of events conducted within the 1-3-7 approach

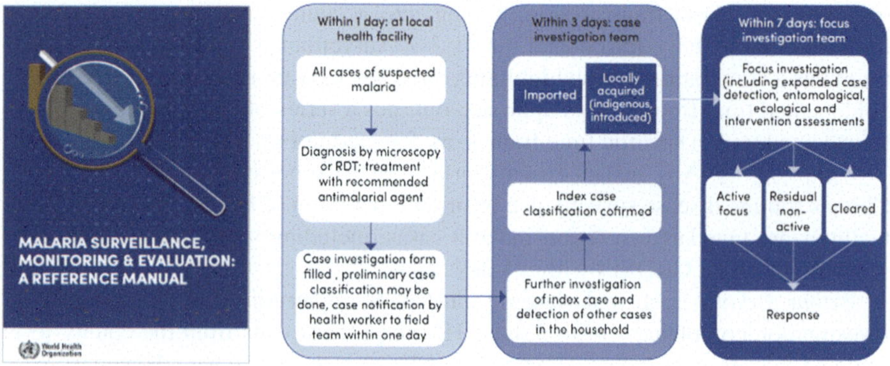

Fig. 1.6 Diagram of 1-3-7 surveillance and response approach presented in the *Malaria Surveillance, Monitoring and Evaluation: A Reference Manual*

transmission risks and associated factors to enable the implementation of precise preventive measures.

The epidemiological and biological evidence supporting the development of the 1-3-7 approach (Cao et al. 2014) is as follows: Firstly, within 1 day: malaria, classified as a class B notifiable infectious disease at the national level, must be reported within 24 h in accordance with China's Law for Prevention and Control of Infectious Diseases. Additionally, the online reporting of cases must be completed within 24 h of diagnosis at any health-care level.

Secondly, within 3 days: patients must receive immediate treatment based on the specific *Plasmodium* species identified. Population interventions will be formulated based on the origins of infection, distinguishing between indigenous and imported cases. Thirdly, within 7 days: considering the life cycle of *Plasmodium vivax*, the predominant species in China, where the parasite completes a full development cycle in vivo in approximately 14 days, the focus of malaria transmission must be addressed within 14 days of infection. The schematic representation of the 1-3-7 approach is depicted in Fig. 1.5.

The 1-3-7 surveillance and response approach serves as a pivotal indicator for assessing the efficacy of key interventions in China's national malaria elimination program. Furthermore, this approach has been adopted in the malaria elimination efforts of various Southeast Asian countries following its inclusion in the global technical guideline for *Malaria Surveillance, Monitoring, and Evaluation: A Reference Manual* published by WHO (WHO 2018) (Fig. 1.6).

1.3 Part 3. Implementation of the 1-3-7 Surveillance and Response Approach in the Jiangsu Provincial Malaria Elimination Program

Adhering strictly to the guidelines outlined in the national document of the 1-3-7 surveillance and response approach, Jiangsu Province bolstered its surveillance and response systems to expedite the malaria elimination efforts. Initially, the province established a comprehensive provincial malaria diagnosis and quality control system, enhancing case identification, reporting, treatment, investigation, and management in alignment with the principles of the 1-3-7 approach. Subsequently, a province-wide blood testing program for fever patients and case-based early warning systems were implemented, encompassing the entire region of Jiangsu Province. These initiatives were supported by the widespread deployment and utilization of RDTs facilitated through the web-based CRDSIS platform.

Moreover, meticulous attention was paid to enhancing the quality of various indicators associated with the 1-3-7 approach within the provincial malaria surveillance and response systems, encompassing aspects such as disease surveillance networks, prompt healthcare-seeking behavior among patients, and capacity-building endeavors. Notably, the establishment of a robust health system and a comprehensive surveillance and response network laid a solid groundwork for the effective implementation of the 1-3-7 approach in Jiangsu Province.

1.3.1 Health Systems in Jiangsu Province

Jiangsu Province comprises 13 prefectures housing a total of 96 counties/districts and 1287 townships (incorporating towns and subdistrict offices). By the end of 2017, the resident population stood at 80.293 million, which included 385,000 individuals from national minority groups such as Mongolian, Hui, Miao, Yi, and Zhuang, constituting 0.5% of the province's total population. In 2017, with a regional gross domestic product (GDP) of RMB 8590.09 billion and a per capita GDP of RMB 107,189, Jiangsu emerged as one of the most dynamic provinces in China in terms of social and economic progress.

As of the end of 2016, Jiangsu boasted a total of over 32,000 health institutions, including 1033 general hospitals at provincial, city (prefecture), and county levels, along with 3701 grassroots health centers and community health service centers. The province also housed approximately 117 disease control institutions at provincial, municipal, and county levels, with a workforce of 517,065 medical and health professionals across all levels. The coverage of the new rural cooperative healthcare scheme exceeded 99% (Commission JH 2016).

1.3.2 Malaria Surveillance and Response Systems in Jiangsu Province

1.3.2.1 Timely Case Reporting

In Jiangsu Province, the establishment of the provincial surveillance and response network has significantly enhanced the efficiency of case identification and reporting across all levels of health-care facilities. This network encompasses activities related to case detection, reporting, epidemiological investigations, and the management of disease clusters conducted by local centers for disease control and prevention (CDCs). When a fever-stricken individual seeks medical attention at various health-care facilities ranging from township to provincial levels, suspected malaria cases undergo blood testing, including microscopy or RDTs. Upon confirmation of a malaria diagnosis, the pertinent details are promptly relayed through CRDSIS (Ma et al. 2006), activating the 1-3-7 approach to prompt rapid responses. Additionally, a mobile phone-based short message service alert system instantly notifies local CDC personnel about the case information, facilitating timely interventions by the local CDC teams.

Question and Answer

5. How can malaria cases be reported post-diagnosis?

Reference answers 5:

Possible methods for reporting include:

1. Utilizing paper-based case reporting.
2. Reporting via telephone.
3. Submitting reports through web-based platforms.
4. Using DHIS2 (District Health Information System II).
5. Implementing electronic reporting systems.
6. Leveraging mobile applications for reporting.
7. Employing email-based reporting mechanisms.
8. Integrating reporting into electronic medical records.
9. Utilizing integrated health information systems for reporting.
10. Directing reports through designated reporting portals.

Proposed discussion time:

- 8 min

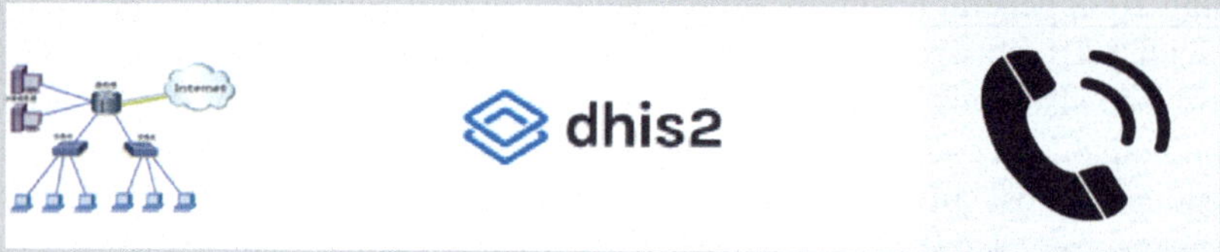

1.3.2.2 Case Investigation and Confirmation Within 3 Days

Following a malaria case report, local CDC staff are required to initiate an investigation within 3 days to confirm the malaria species and ascertain the origins of the infection. The county-level CDC, where the case is initially reported, is responsible for confirming all malaria cases and conducting investigations into the infectious origins to determine whether the case is indigenous or imported. Based on this distinction, appropriate treatment and containment measures must be promptly implemented. To ensure effective case investigation within this time frame, it is crucial to address three key elements: WHO, WHEN, and WHAT. Local county or municipal CDCs, where the malaria case is reported, are mandated to complete the case investigation within 3 days. By the end of this period, CDC personnel must finalize the investigation and complete a survey questionnaire detailing essential information about the malaria case, such as health-seeking behavior, antimalarial treatment, travel history, illness history, infection sources, follow-up procedures, date of patients' return to China, and accompanying workers or relatives.

Question and Answer

6. How should malaria cases be reported post-diagnosis?

Reference answers 6:

- Malaria YES/NOT?
- How to exclude?
- The major diagnostic tools: RDT/Microscopy/PCR?

Proposed discussion time:

- 5 min

Finally, all the pertinent investigation details regarding the malaria case must be promptly uploaded to the web-based CRDSIS platform within 3 days.

Question and Answer

7. How to differentiate between local and imported malaria infections?

Reference answers 7:

It needs the following evidences:

- Local or imported cases?
- Case investigation?
- Epidemiological survey?
- Molecular evidence?

Proposed discussion time:

- 5 min

1.3.2.3 Focus Investigation and Response Activities Within 7 Days

The focus investigation must be promptly initiated to address potential local malaria transmission. In cases where local transmission is either possible or confirmed, targeted actions should be promptly implemented to detect and prevent further infections. All response activities aimed at reducing the risk of onward transmission must be completed within 7 days by the county CDC staff. When conducting focus response activities in Jiangsu Province, it is essential to document the key elements: WHO, WHEN, and WHAT.

Regarding WHO, local county or municipal CDCs in the vicinity of the malaria case's residence are responsible for carrying out focus disposals. As for WHEN, all information related to focus investigations and disposals must be uploaded to the web-based CRDSIS within a 7-day time frame. In terms of WHAT, the local CDC staff should complete a foci investigation questionnaire encompassing essential details such as entomology surveys, foci classification, foci disposal (RACD), targeted MDA, vector control measures, and health education initiatives.

Question and Answer

8. How to implement focus/foci investigation after case confirmation?

Reference answers 8:

Transmission risk will be assessed through epidemiology and entomology survey.

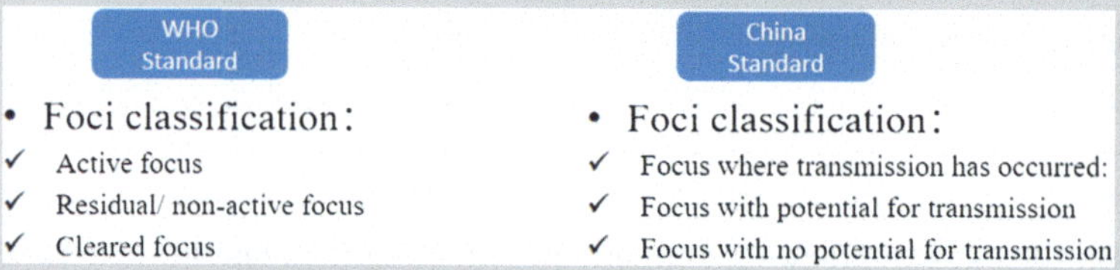

Proposed discussion time:

– 5 min

9. How to carry out focus/foci disposal effectively?

Reference answers 9:

Measures	Focus with occurred transmission	Focus with transmission risk	Focus without transmission risk
RACD	√		
Targeted MDA	√		
Vector control (IRS)	√	√	
Health education	√	√	√

Proposed discussion time:

– 5 min

1.3.3 *Innovative Approach to Health Education for Accessing Health-Care Services by Patients*

Under the guidance of the Health Administrative Department and in conjunction with the annual public awareness activities for the National Malaria Day on April 26, various health education initiatives were undertaken in all endemic areas of Jiangsu Province. These initiatives included the dissemination of health education materials such as slogans, leaflets, posters, promotional banners, audiovisual broadcasts, and traditional paper folding techniques aimed at local residents and high-risk populations. The educational campaigns provided information on malaria prevention and control. Additionally, collaborative multisectoral meetings were organized to share information on malaria control through newspapers, radio, television, and other communication channels. In recent years, emerging online platforms such as Douyin (TikTok), WeChat, and Weibo, which are highly popular in China, have been utilized to disseminate extensive information on malaria control (Fig. 1.7).

1.3.4 *Implementing Malaria Technical Training Courses for All Levels of Health-Care Facilities*

In Jiangsu Province, a range of malaria training programs and initiatives have been carried out for health-care facilities at all levels. These initiatives include training on RDT application and management, aimed at enhancing the awareness and proficiency of health-care providers in malaria diagnosis and treatment.

Moreover, technical posters, such as Standard Operating Procedures (SOP) for microscopy and RDT, have been displayed on hospital walls, and mugs containing

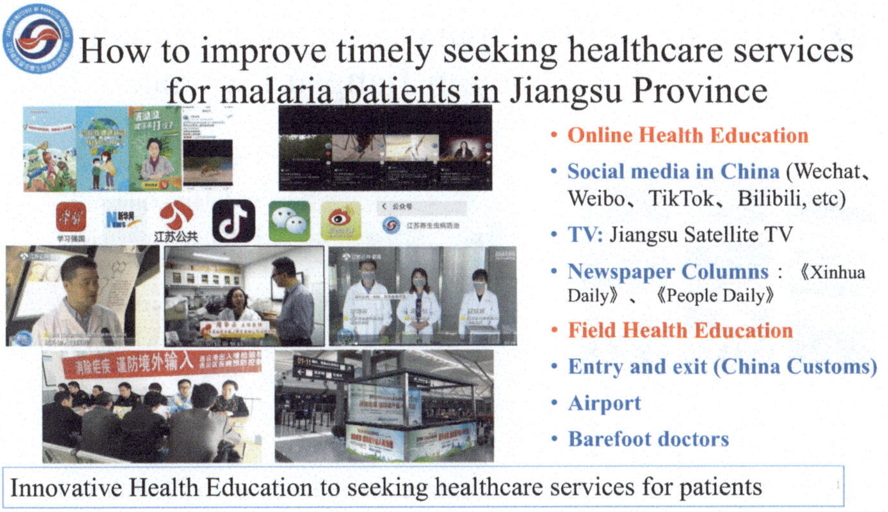

Fig. 1.7 Innovative health education to improve health-care seeking of patients

information on malaria control have been distributed to local residents. These educational materials with technical content are provided to local CDCs and hospitals to enhance the technical capabilities of health-care facilities at the local level (Fig. 1.8).

1.3.5 Conducting Tabletop Exercises to Enhance the Regulation of Focal/Foci Disposal

The understanding of the 1-3-7 approach among health-care personnels at grassroots CDCs in Jiangsu Province was initially limited. However, tabletop exercises focusing on the implementation of the 1-3-7 approach proved to be more effective in improving the comprehension of the entire procedure among grassroots personnel compared to traditional classroom-style training. Consequently, tabletop exercises on the implementation of the 1-3-7 approach have been widely conducted in the endemic counties of Jiangsu Province.

1.3.6 Quality Control of the 1-3-7 Approach

The Jiangsu Institute of Parasitic Diseases (JIPD), a provincial-level professional organization dedicated to the prevention and control of parasitic diseases, assumed responsibility for ensuring the quality of the 1-3-7 approach implementation. Various departments within JIPD, such as the Department of Malaria Control, Information and Health Education Center, Central Laboratory, and other relevant

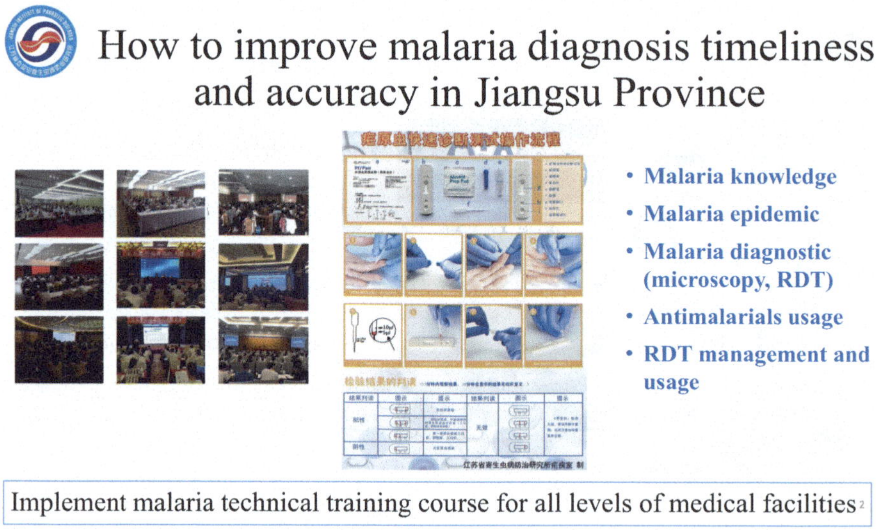

Fig. 1.8 Implementation of malaria technical training course for all levels of medical facilities

divisions, were actively engaged in malaria control activities. These activities included aiding the Provincial Health and Family Planning Commission in formulating malaria prevention plans and technical strategies, offering technical guidance and professional training, monitoring epidemic trends, managing reported cases, conducting supervision and quality assessments, coordinating investigations and research, procuring and distributing disease-testing equipment and antimalarial drugs, as well as creating and disseminating health education materials.

To maintain quality control of the 1-3-7 approach during the malaria elimination phase, JIPD implemented various activities. These activities encompassed quality control measures for malaria diagnosis at reference laboratories, regular reviews of online reported cases, statistical analysis of malaria epidemic trends, on-site epidemiological investigations, vector surveillance and monitoring, experimental research on mosquito vectors, development of educational materials on malaria prevention, and the upkeep of a provincial travel malaria information website containing relevant prevention and health education resources.

1.3.7 Networking for Malaria Surveillance and Response Systems

Apart from the surveillance and response initiatives spearheaded by JIPD at the provincial level, all institutions at the municipal and county levels actively participate in malaria surveillance and response efforts.

To begin with, each of the 13 municipal CDCs in Jiangsu Province houses specialized departments tasked with overseeing, inspecting, evaluating, and ensuring the quality of malaria control activities within their respective jurisdictions. These departments collaborate with JIPD to conduct various quality control measures. Additionally, all 96 county-level (city-level, district-level) CDCs in Jiangsu Province have dedicated departments and personnel responsible for conducting case reviews, epidemiological investigations, managing epidemic hot spots, guiding townships in implementing blood tests for patients with "three fevers," ensuring quality control, training grassroots malaria control staff, collecting and reporting pertinent malaria control data, and supporting higher-level institutions in executing diverse malaria control initiatives.

Furthermore, the Jiangsu Entry-Exit Inspection and Quarantine Bureau has established 17 International Travel Health Care Centers, all of which are equipped to conduct malaria case screenings and parasite detection as per the requirements for individuals returning from overseas and passing through customs.

Finally, medical institutions, hospitals, and health centers at all levels are entrusted with diagnosing, reporting, and treating malaria cases while supporting CDCs in conducting epidemiological investigations and case sampling. Building upon the completion of blood tests for patients with "three fevers," including those with malaria, suspected malaria, and fevers of unknown origin, grassroots health centers and community health service centers collaboratively engage in numerous activities aimed at malaria elimination. These activities encompass investigations and monitoring, community health education and promotion, as well as the analysis of epidemic data and management of epidemic hot spots. Village clinics also play a crucial role in fulfilling various malaria control and monitoring tasks assigned by higher-level institutions. As a result, a relatively robust network system for malaria surveillance and response has been successfully established in the province.

1.4 Part 4. Assessment of the 1-3-7 Approach Effectiveness in Jiangsu Province

Between 2001 and 2020, a total of 9879 malaria cases were reported in Jiangsu Province (Fig. 1.9). The majority of cases reported during this period were indigenous cases, with 69.02% (4864 cases) originating locally, while 22.92% (1615 cases) were imported from other provinces within China and 8.06% (568 cases) originated from other countries. However, from 2011 to 2020, only 13 indigenous vivax malaria cases were reported in Jiangsu Province, with 2786 cases being imported from other countries. Notably, all 13 indigenous cases were reported in 2011.

Following the initiation of the 1-3-7 surveillance approach in 2012, there was a significant shift in the patterns of malaria cases. In 2012, indigenous vivax malaria cases dropped to zero, and since then, all malaria cases in Jiangsu Province were imported from abroad. Over the past decade, out of 91 severe malaria cases recorded, there were eight malaria-related deaths, all of which were linked to imported malaria cases. No any case of introduced malaria was detected in Jiangsu Province.

Among the sources of imported malaria cases from 2012 to 2020, four cases were linked to infections through blood transfusions from imported cases abroad, while 2419 cases were individuals returning from countries in Africa, Southeast Asia, and South America. The majority of these cases originated from Equatorial Guinea (532 cases, 21.96%), Angola (526 cases, 21.71%), Nigeria (272 cases, 11.23%), Republic of Congo (138 cases, 5.69%), and Cameroon (114 cases, 4.71%), accounting for 65.29% (1582 cases) of all imported cases.

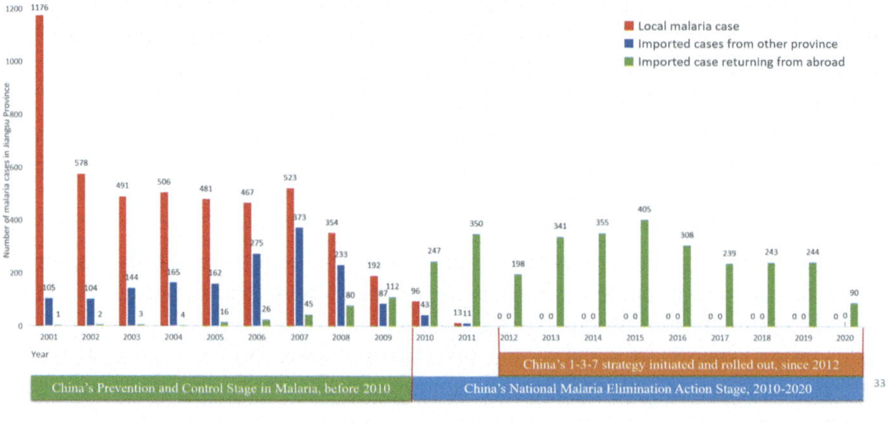

Fig. 1.9 Malaria epidemiological trends in Jiangsu Province

1.4.1 Indicators of 1-3-7 Approach Implementation in Jiangsu Province

In Jiangsu Province, professionals from CDCs at all levels have introduced innovative training methods, such as tabletop exercises for addressing malaria hot spots. Since the implementation of the 1-3-7 approach in 2012, all malaria cases have been promptly reported via the web-based CRDSIS system, with local medical facility staff completing the "Reporting Card for Infectious Diseases" within 1 day or 24 h, achieving a 100% reporting rate. Additionally, over 98% of malaria cases have undergone individual epidemiological investigations conducted by local CDC staff at the county level within 3 days, following the guidelines outlined in the *Protocol on Epidemiological Survey of Malaria Cases*. Regarding hot spot management, more than 98% of foci have been addressed within 7 days, as indicated in Table 1.2.

However, the onset of the COVID-19 pandemic had an impact on these operations, leading to a decrease in the proportion of foci investigated within 7 days, with the rate dropping to 90% in 2020.

1.4.2 Shrinking Malaria Maps Confirmed by County-Level Assessment in Jiangsu Province from 2010 to 2020

Since 2012, a county-level assessment on malaria elimination progress was caried out every year in Jiangsu Province. A total of 100 counties in Jiangsu province were individually monitored and assessed for malaria elimination. As a result, Sheyang

Table 1.2 Indicators of the "1-3-7" approach in Jiangsu Province from 2012 to 2020

	Case detection and notification			Case investigation		Focus investigation and action	
Year	Number of malaria cases	Number of case reporting within 1 day	Proportion of case reporting within 1 day	Number of case investigation within 3 days	Proportion of case investigation within 3 days	Number of foci investigation and action within 7 days	Proportion of foci investigation and action within 7 days
2012	198	198	100.00%	193	98.97%	191	96.46%
2013	341	341	100.00%	341	100.00%	341	100.00%
2014	355	355	100.00%	355	100.00%	355	100.00%
2015	405	405	100.00%	405	100.00%	405	100.00%
2016	308	308	100.00%	308	100.00%	308	100.00%
2017	239	239	100.00%	231	97.91%	223	93.31%
2018	243	243	100.00%	242	99.59%	240	98.77%
2019	244	244	100.00%	244	100.00%	238	97.54%
2020	90	90	100.00%	90	100.00%	81	90%
Total	2423	2423	100.00%	2409	99.42%	2382	98.31%

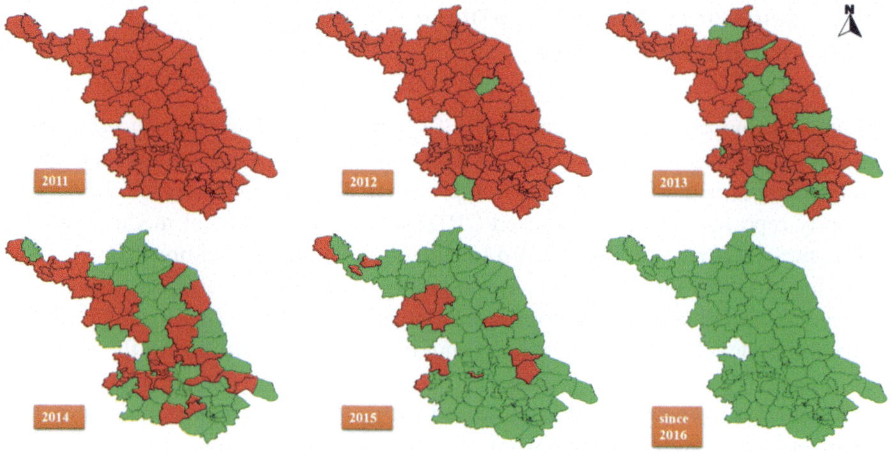

Fig. 1.10 Maps showing malaria elimination progress in Jiangsu Province from 2010 to 2020

County and Liyang County firstly reached the criteria of malaria elimination and passed the county-level assessment of malaria free. By the end of 2016, all of 100 counties in Jiangsu Province passed county-level assessment. In 2017, all of 13 prefectural cities in Jiangsu Province passed the municipal-level assessment of malaria elimination, therefore whole province achieved the goal of eliminating malaria (Fig. 1.10).

1.5 Part 5. Challenges and Solutions to Implement the 1-3-7 Approach in Jiangsu Province

As efforts progress toward eliminating malaria, significant challenges have surfaced in maintaining robust surveillance systems and swiftly executing the 1-3-7 approach during both the elimination and post-elimination phases. Moreover, the issue of preventing imported malaria cases from overseas has gained prominence. Alongside the increasing global economic integration facilitated by initiatives like the "Belt and Road," there has been a noticeable surge in individuals participating in work, travel, business ventures, and international exchanges abroad. This rise in international mobility inherently escalates the risk of imported mosquito-borne infectious diseases, including malaria.

In anticipation of these hurdles, consultations were arranged among experts from the 13 municipal centers for disease control and prevention (CDCs) across the province. In 2017, a comprehensive report outlining the new challenges encountered and the corresponding solutions devised was compiled. This report stands as a valuable asset that can be shared with regions currently undergoing malaria elimination or transitioning into the post-elimination phase.

Question and Answer

10. Possible challenges and measures to implement the 1-3-7 approach in your country?

Reference answers 10:

Every country faces unique challenges when implementing the 1-3-7 approach in combating diseases like malaria. However, there are some common obstacles and corresponding measures that are often encountered:

Challenges:

- Resource constraints
- Awareness deficit
- Geographical barriers
- Health-care system weaknesses
- ....

Measures:

- Enhanced funding
- Community engagement
- Utilization of technology
- Capacity development
- Emergency response planning
- ....

Proposed discussion time:

- 8 min

1.5.1 Public Health Management Assurance

As Jiangsu Province advances in malaria elimination, preventing the reintroduction of malaria becomes a key focus during the post-elimination phase. This phase requires a heightened emphasis on strengthening activities related to sensitive surveillance and immediate responses. However, a significant challenge arises due to a shortage of professionals engaged in surveillance and response efforts.

Furthermore, insufficient funding for preventing the reintroduction of malaria, especially at the grassroots level, presents a significant concern. Additional challenges arise from a lack of policy backing, inadequate attention from leaders, and deficiencies in laboratory and clinical personnel. These factors contribute to further hurdles, including a lack of awareness concerning malaria diagnosis and treatment in medical facilities.

1.5.2 Patient Healthcare-Seeking Behavior and Diagnosis and Treatment by Medical Facilities

In medical settings, the majority of imported cases are swiftly diagnosed, with fewer than one-sixth of patients remaining undiagnosed after 3 days. Consequently, in instances of persistent fever, local medical practitioners should exercise caution and inquire about the patient's travel history to identify suspected malaria cases. Furthermore, village doctors and township health workers should promptly refer suspected malaria patients to higher-level health facilities for further evaluation and treatment.

The delay in seeking health care, diagnosis, and treatment for malaria is linked to an increased risk of severe illness or mortality. Therefore, there is a pressing need to enhance the healthcare-seeking behavior of malaria patients and the diagnostic skills of health-care providers. In Jiangsu Province, a deficiency in malaria diagnostic capacity was noted, particularly concerning blood smear microscopy at the township and village levels. The training and use of RDTs in Jiangsu Province have improved health-care accessibility for malaria patients, proving to be an effective strategy in reducing delayed diagnoses among individuals with malaria.

1.5.3 Case Inquiry and Focus Disposal

Since early 2012, the nationwide adoption of the 1-3-7 surveillance and response approach has been crucial in identifying, treating, and promptly containing individual malaria cases while preventing transmission. In malaria elimination areas such as Jiangsu Province, monitoring and assessing malaria case investigations can significantly improve program effectiveness, bringing it to the required level for successful elimination. Regularly organizing provincial-level parasitic diagnostic skills competitions in Jiangsu Province helps sustain diagnostic capabilities and enhances the proficiency of microscopy examiners in local hospitals and CDCs, providing strong technical support for malaria elimination endeavors. Enhancing laboratory diagnostic capacities in local hospitals, ensuring the consistent treatment of imported malaria cases, and reducing severe outcomes and fatalities are vital measures that can enhance the overall response to malaria in the area.

The provincial malaria surveillance and response network cover case identification and reporting at all levels of medical facilities, alongside epidemiological investigations and focus management at CDCs (Fig. 1.11) (Cao et al. 2022). Currently, the laboratory departments of over 2170 medical institutions in the province can carry out *Plasmodium* spp. detection, with around 5000 laboratory staff members having undergone training at county, city, and provincial levels for

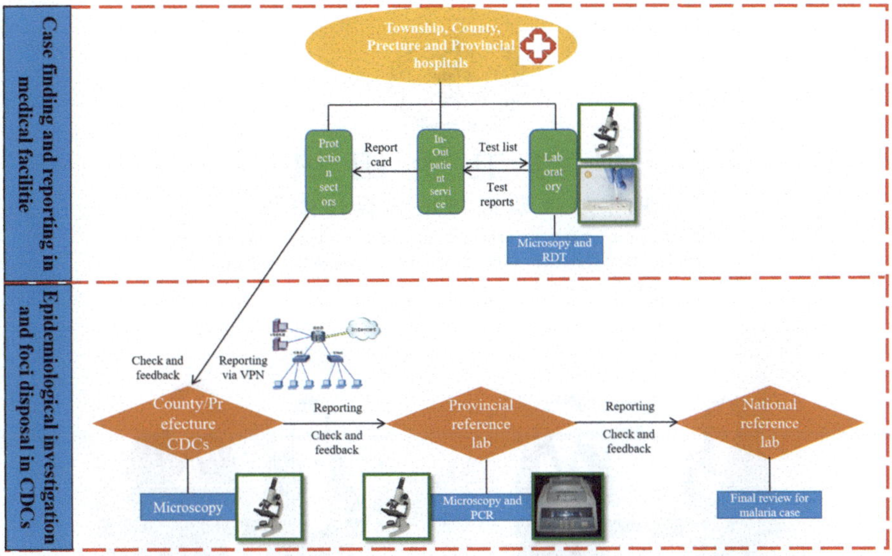

Fig. 1.11 Malaria surveillance and response network in Jiangsu Province

microscopic examination of *Plasmodium* spp. Apart from *Plasmodium* spp. detection, medical institutions at each level have gradually introduced RDT on a trial basis and have advocated for RDT usage for patients showing "three fevers" since 2013, thereby enhancing *Plasmodium* spp. detection capabilities by combining these two methods. Any malaria cases identified by medical institutions at any level are reported through the epidemic reporting system within 24 h. Results are reviewed, and any duplicates are eliminated after evaluation by county-level CDC staff. When a patient with a fever visits a hospital, suspected cases presenting "three fever" undergo blood tests and/or RDT. Upon confirmation, relevant information on the malaria case is reported through the web-based CRDSIS, triggering the commencement of the 1-3-7 approach for a swift and coordinated response.

In 2016, JIPD was designated as a WHO Collaborating Centre for Research and Training on Malaria Elimination. This designation tasks the WHO Collaborating Center with the responsibility of gathering and formulating strategies and technologies relevant to malaria elimination, as well as conducting training and scientific research to support malaria elimination efforts. Utilizing its role as a World Health Organization Collaboration Centre, JIPD is dedicated to providing continuous technical support for global malaria elimination initiatives and actively engaging in the establishment of a unified global health community (Fig. 1.12).

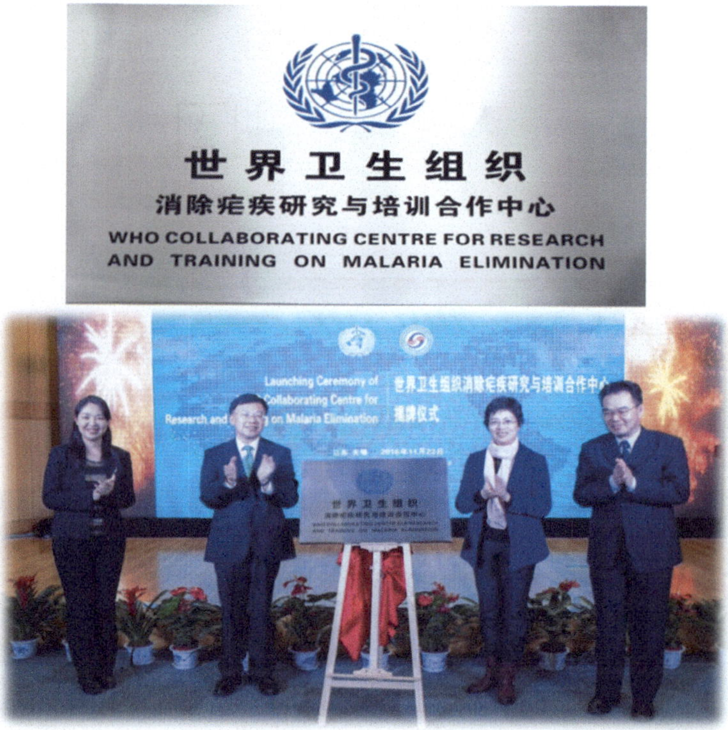

Fig. 1.12 JIPD designated as a WHO Collaborating Centre for Research and Training on Malaria Elimination in October, 2016

Acknowledgments This work was supported by the Bill & Melinda Gates Foundation (No. INV-018913).

References

Bastaki H, Carter J, Marston L, Cassell J, Rait G (2018) Time delays in the diagnosis and treatment of malaria in non-endemic countries: a systematic review. Travel Med Infect Dis 21:21–27

Cao J, Zhou SS, Zhou HY, Yu YB, Tang LH, Gao Q (2013) Malaria from control to elimination in China: transition of goal, strategy and interventions. Zhongguo Xue Xi Chong Bing Fang Zhi Za Zhi 25:439–443

Cao J, Sturrock HJ, Cotter C, Zhou S, Zhou H, Liu Y, Tang L, Gosling RD, Feachem RG, Gao Q (2014) Communicating and monitoring surveillance and response activities for malaria elimination: China's "1-3-7" strategy. PLoS Med 11:e1001642

Cao Y, Lu G, Cotter C, Wang W, Yang M, Liu Y, Liang C, Zhou H, Lu Y, Yan J, Zhu G, Cao J (2022) Improving the surveillance and response system to achieve and maintain malaria elimination: a retrospective analysis in Jiangsu Province, China. Infect Dis Poverty 11(1):20.

Jiangsu Health Commission (2016). Jiangsu Health Yearbook. Science and Technology Literature Press, Beijing

Feng J, Zhang L, Huang F, Yin JH, Tu H, Xia ZG, Zhou SS, Xiao N, Zhou XN (2018) Ready for malaria elimination: zero indigenous case reported in the People's Republic of China. Malar J 17:315

Lei ZL, Wang LY (2012) Control situation and primary task of key parasitic diseases in China. Zhongguo Ji Sheng Chong Xue Yu Ji Sheng Chong Bing Za Zhi 30:1–5

Ma JQ, Wang LP, Qi XP, Shi XM, Yang GH (2006) The conceptual model of the automatic early-warning system of infectious diseases monitoring based on direct network reporting system. Dis Surveill 21(12):679–682

Tang LH (1999) Achievements of malaria control and research in China. Zhongguo Ji Sheng Chong Xue Yu Ji Sheng Chong Bing Za Zhi 17:257

WHO (2015) WHO: Global Technical Strategy for Malaria 2016–2030. WHO, Geneva

WHO (2017) WHO: a framework for malaria elimination. WHO, Geneva

WHO (2018) WHO: Malaria surveillance, monitoring & evaluation: a reference manual. WHO, Geneva

WHO (2020) WHO: World Malaria Report 2020. WHO, Geneva, p 299

Zhou SS, Wang Y, Xia ZG (2011) Malaria situation in the People's Republic of China in 2009. Zhongguo Ji Sheng Chong Xue Yu Ji Sheng Chong Bing Za Zhi 29:1–3

Zhou HY, Cao J, Wang WM, Liu YB, Cao YY, Gao Q (2013) Epidemiological analysis of malaria prevalence in Jiangsu Province in 2011. Zhongguo Xue Xi Chong Bing Fang Zhi Za Zhi 25:31–35

Chapter 2
Malaria Along International Border in Yunnan of China, 2003–2020: A Case Study of Border Malaria Control and Elimination

Hui Liu, Cang-Lin Zhang, Qi-Yan Chen, Yao-Wu Zhou, and Jian-Wei Xu

Abbreviations

ACT	Artemisinin-based combination therapy
API	Annual parasite incidence
CDC	Centers for Disease Control and Prevention
EHO	Ethnic Health Organizations
GMS	Great Mekong Subregion
HPA	Health poverty action
IRS	Indoor residual spraying
IDP	Internal displaced person
KR2	Kachin Special Region II
LLINs	Long-lasting insecticide impregnated bed nets
MDA	Mass drug administration
MDT	Mean distance traveled
MMRR	Mosquito mark-release-recapture
NGO	Nongovernmental organization
PCR	Polymerase chain reaction
RDTs	Rapid diagnostic tests
RACD	Reactive case detection
WHO	World Health Organization
YIPD	Yunnan Institute of Parasitic Diseases

Introduction

Participants can use the module to think their own country's issue of border malaria. Due to its inclusion of answers to many exercises, it should not be provided before the end.

Participants should be advised to read the following documents before and during the course:

H. Liu (✉) · C.-L. Zhang · Q.-Y. Chen · Y.-W. Zhou · J.-W. Xu
Yunnan Institute of Parasitic Diseases, Puer, Yunnan, People's Republic of China

X.-N. Zhou, J.-H. Yin (eds.), *Malaria Control and Elimination in China*,
https://doi.org/10.1007/978-981-97-8719-7_2

- Eliminating malaria. Geneva: World Health Organization, 2016.
- A framework for malaria elimination. Geneva: World Health Organization, 2017.
- WHO guidelines for malaria. Geneva: World Health Organization, 2023.

Learning Objectives
By the end of this course, wish that you will be able to:

1. Answer these questions that can be applied, from the malaria hyperendemicity to control, and finally elimination and prevention of malaria reintroduction.

2.1 Information 1: Challenges of Border Malaria Control and Elimination

2.1.1 Objective

By the end of this chapter, participants can be able to understand their main challenges of border malaria control and elimination in their country.

2.1.2 Background of Border Malaria in Yunnan

Yunnan, located in Southwestern China and part of the Greater Mekong Subregion (GMS), is one of only two provinces in China where *Plasmodium falciparum* is endemic after 2000. The province has a border of 4060 km with Myanmar, Lao PDR, and Vietnam. Yunnan is mountainous, with an altitude of 76.4 m to 6740 m, and the climate ranges from tropical to cold. The border and low altitude areas are the main areas where malaria is prevalent. It has a population of 48 million and is comprised of 26 ethnic groups. More than 80% of people in the region still have a risk of malaria infection (Xu and Liu 1997). The neighboring country of Myanmar bears the highest malaria burden and ranks 31st among countries with the highest malaria burden globally. Thirteen indigenous minorities reside on both sides across the international border. Yunnan has 5 national level and 12 provincial level border ports, and 226 unofficial border crossing points, and there are no natural or artificial barriers along the international border. In Yunnan's border areas where mosquito vectors are highly efficient in terms of malaria transmission capacity, the transmission season is long or year-round, poor communities with overall development, marginalized populations with insufficient health service coverage, and weak health systems, as well as neighboring areas with civil unrest, illegal cross-border flows, high border burdens, and intense cross-border population movements, malaria transmission is particularly difficult to stop. Each of these factors will reduce the feasibility of eliminating malaria.

2.1.3 *Main Challenges in Border Malaria Elimination in Yunnan*

1. Yunnan shares a long border of 4060 km with three malaria endemic countries: Myanmar, Lao PDR, and Vietnam.
2. The diversity in vector species and the tremendous spatial heterogeneity in distribution patterns.
3. The border areas of Yunnan and neighboring counties were originally hyperendemic.
4. Yunnan border has 13 indigenous ethnic minorities living across the international border which are politically, economically, culturally, and geographically marginalized.
5. Border regions experience a heavy population flow, and the mobile and displaced populations increase the risk of infection as they are exposed to new environments with new vectors and malaria ecologies.
6. Yunnan's international borders have almost no natural and artificial barriers.
7. Some border regions are densely forested, which increases malaria transmission and serves as reservoirs of malaria parasites.

   Notes: According to the WHO recommendation on malaria program phases and milestones on the path to malaria elimination, the malaria control and elimination program of Yunnan province from hyperendemicity to elimination during 2003 to 2013 was divided into three phases, namely control (2003–2013), elimination (2014–2016), and reintroduction prevention (2017–2020).

2.1.4 *Exercise*

Question and Answer
1. Is there any border malaria problem in your country? What are the main challenges of malaria elimination in your country?

(As an opening question)
Reference answer:

- For example: situation of border area in Yunnan.

Recommended discussion time:

- 5–10 min

2.2 Information 2: Reduction of Malaria Burden

2.2.1 Objective

By the end of this part, learners should know what strategy can be used to reduce malaria burden rapidly down to the elimination stage.

2.2.2 Goal and Strategy

The goal of this phase is to reduce malaria burden significantly and make effort to lower annual parasite incidence (API) forward to elimination (API < 1 per 10,000 person-years). The strategies included:

1. Upgrading information collection and reporting system to reduce underreported malaria cases. The local health facilities are requested to report both confirmed and suspected malaria cases within 24 h using the web-based China Information System for Disease Control and Prevention (CISDCP) (Ma et al. 2006; Yang et al. 2011).
2. Using integrated control interventions including standard treatment for lab-confirmed malaria cases, radical treatment for *vivax* malaria and *ovale* malaria cases, presumptive treatment for suspected malaria cases and preventive treatment for people as high risks, as well as vector control with indoor residual spraying (IRS) with insecticides and use insecticide-treated bed nets (Xu et al. 2021a).
3. Following stratification of malaria prevalence and infection risk, interventions of "locally-oriented, burden-oriented, special strategy for special area" were conducted.

2.2.3 Exercise

Question and Answer

2. What conditions are suitable to use IRS?

Reference answer:

1. IRS depends on the availability of the national vector control services, as well as sufficient human, financial, and logistical resources, including skilled spraying teams, storage and transport facilities, and spraying equipment. There should be clear human resource polices (e.g., whether sprayers should be temporary workers or permanent staff?) and should ensure effective administration to manage these resources.

2. Due to the fact that it usually requires several years of consecutive rounds of IRS to achieve and sustain the full potential of this intervention, its adoption requires a medium- to long-term financial and political commitment from local authorities, funding partners, and national programs to achieve it.
3. Based on accurate entomological and epidemiological information plan, an IRS that involves insecticide resistance, vector identification and biomics, including their feeding and resting behavior as well as transmission dynamics (rhythm and intensity). Only insecticides that are susceptible to vector should be used. The factor of insecticide resistance within and near the target area determines the kind of insecticides for procurement. The decision should be consistent with the national resistance management policy and compared with it. This must be completed as early as possible, as procurement delays are common.
4. The geographical reconnaissance determined the number, nature, and location, and access of spraying sites.
5. Most vector populations feed and rest indoors.
6. People who mainly sleep indoors at night.
7. One or two rounds of IRS can be used annually to protect the transmission patterns of malaria among the population.
8. Most structures are suitable for spraying.

Recommended discussion time:

- 20–30 min.

3. What are the usage conditions for LLINs?
Reference answer:

1. Due to the large volume of mosquito nets, it is necessary to consider their storage and transport to target communities. It is necessary to estimate the time of procurement, storage, and transportation, in order to provide sufficient numbers of LLINs when and where they are needed.
2. To provide LLINs freely to target communities without gap in the supply chain. Due to migration, extra nets may be required after 1 year and should be replaced after 3 years or through continuous channels.
3. Distribution of LLINs should be based mainly on malaria prevalence and demographic information. A decision should be taken at an early stage about how many nets should be delivered per capita and how many per household, depending on whether there are one, two, or up to ten inhabitants. The size, color, strength, etc. should be decided.
4. Resistance to many insecticides (e.g., pyrethroids) poses a serious threat to the control of all types of malaria vectors and requires continuous monitor-

ing. Some information indicates that the effect of LLINs may be reduced in areas with vector resistance, but further evaluation of the impact of resistance is necessary.

Recommended discussion time:

- 20–30 min

4. What is the term of mass drug adminstration (MDA)? Which factors should be considered if primaquine is used in MDA?

Reference answer:

MDA: At the same time, often at repeated intervals, antimalarial treatment is administered to defined population or every person living in a defined geographical area (excluding people with contraindication to this drug).

If primaquine is used in MDA, the following factors will be considered:

1. In relation to the safety issue: There are good reasons to include a single dose of primaquine. If your country already uses it on a large scale, it should be fine. Otherwise, 0.25 mg/kg could be an option to prevent transmission. While the MDA takes place, a qualified clinician should be available, rapid evacuation for blood transfusion should be possible, if there is a concern that one of the dangerous types of G6PT deficiency is prevalent.
2. Previous experiences do not point to a clear benefit. MDA may result in an important short-term reduction in the parasite reservoir but has little impact on transmission rates over time.
3. Primaquine, which was often employed in MDA, carries a risk of life-threatening hemolysis in people who have the genetic trait of glucose-6-phosphate dehydrogenase deficiency, which is particularly prevalent in malaria-endemic regions.
4. The indiscriminate use of medicines in MDA increases the risk of the parasite developing drug resistance.

Recommended discussion time:

- 20–30 min

2.3 Information 3: Malaria Elimination

2.3.1 Objective

By the end of this part, learners should know how to interrupt malaria transmission?

The WHO recommends that in areas where the first program reorientation has been achieved, as well as in areas where health facility data shows an annual parasite incidence (API) of less than 1 case per 1000 people at risk, equal to less than

100 new cases per year in an area with a population of 100,000. In China, the smallest unit for elimination is in a county with a population of one million in most parts. China malaria elimination program recommends that elimination phase starts after the API of less than 0.1 infections per 1000 people. The milestone depends on where there are human resources in the areas being considered for elimination. The recent successful efforts to eliminate malaria have been initiated by countries where the total nationwide malaria caseload was ≤1000 per year (e.g., China reaches the goal in 2009).

The mid-population of a border county in Yunnan is around 300,000 people. Considering the high risk of infection in the border areas, Yunnan also reorientated its program toward elimination after achieving an API of less than 0.1 infections per 1000 people. By 2013, the overall API was reduced to 0.039 per 1000 person years in the 25 border counties. Only 49 indigenous malaria cases were reported. The API of indigenous infections was much less than 0.1 infections per 1000 people in every county. All 25 border counties, also the whole Yunnan, reorientated to elimination program since 2014.

2.3.2 Goal and Strategy

1. The goal of this phase is completely to interrupt malaria transmission to achieve zero indigenous acquired cases in 25 border counties. Meanwhile, cross-border collaboration was reemphasized to reduce the imported malaria and decrease the risk of infection.
2. The strategy in general of "clearing parasite reservoirs, tracking infectious sources" were conducted by intensive surveillances, epidemiological investigations, and rapid public health responses. And decision-making establishing a reference laboratory system to validate the parasitic diagnosis of malaria.

2.3.3 Exercise

Question and Answer

5. When a malaria program can be reorientated from pre-elimination to elimination? What is a suitable unit for elimination? Why?

(As an opening question)

Reference answer:

- Recommended discussion time: 5–10 min.
- Key points of answers:

Malaria programme phases and milestones on the path to malaria elimination[a]

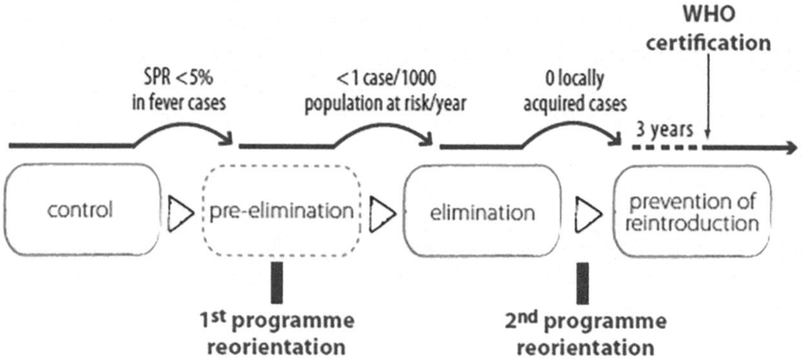

SPR: slide or rapid diagnostic test positivity rate.

[a] These milestones are indicative only: in practice, the transitions will depend on the malaria burden that a programme can realistically handle (including case notification, case investigation, etc.).

- As shown in this figure, the WHO recommends that a malaria program can be reorientated from pre-elimination to elimination after the API was reduced to <1/1000 person years. The WHO also recommends that the smallest unit for malaria elimination is a district with at least a population of 100,000 people. Therefore, the WHO recommended reorientation from pre-elimination to elimination is based on a population size of 100,000 people. Where the elimination phase starts in areas where the pre-elimination reorientation has been achieved, and where health facility data show a malaria incidence of less than 1 infection per 1000 people at risk per year, equal to less than 100 new cases per year in a district with a population of 100,000 people or less than 3 malaria cases per response team.
- In China, a county is selected as a unit for malaria elimination. Based on the average population of a county with one response team is about one million in China. The reorientation from pre-elimination to elimination was nationally recommended after the API < 1/10000 person years.
- Yunnan is a mountainous province with a much lower population density but a large land area. The media population size of a county is about 350,000 that are much less than the average size of one million population; however, most population of Yunnan is difficult to access due to the landform and inconvenient transportation. As the national request across China, a county is also defined as unit of malaria elimination, and the pre-elimination to elimination was also reorientated after the API < 1/10,000 person years. However, the reduced size of population and number of malaria cases do not mean any reduced work burden because of the difficult accessibility to communities and the threats from neighboring countries.

6. According to the data in Table 2.1, **what stage of malaria program in each county of 25 Yunnan's border counties in 2013 based on the WHO's standard and China's standard, respectively?**

Reference answer:

– 25 Yunnan's border counties are the stage of malaria elimination.

Recommended time:

– 5 min

As conclusion, summarize the main points in the learning unit and go through the learning objectives with the participants to confirm that they were met. Alternatively, ask three or more participants state the main lessons they have learned in this unit.

Table 2.1 Malaria burden of Yunnan 25 border counties in 2013

County	No. of cases	No. of indigenous	No. of population	API/10000	API/10,000 of indigenous
Fugong	4	1	102,170	0.39	0.10
Gongshan	1	–	39,475	0.25	0
Lushui	6	–	179,959	0.33	0
Tenchong	149	4	745,378	2.0	0.05
Longling	14	2	309,994	0.45	0.06
Yingjiang	72	18	301,751	2.39	0.60
Ruili	133	3	191,569	6.94	0.16
Luxi	25	5	69,662	3.59	0.72
Longchuan	14	–	208,985	0.67	0
Cangyuan	6	4	197,374	0.3	0.20
Gengma	11	9	363,633	0.3	0.25
Zhenkang	3	–	201,206	0.15	0
Lancang	4	–	523,623	0.08	0
Menglian	9	–	127,713	0.7	0
Ximeng	2	–	92,882	0.22	0
Menghai	1	–	348,308	0.03	0
Jinghong	5	–	510,851	0.1	0
Mengla	8	1	232,205	0.34	0.04
Jiangcheng	5	2	104,492	0.48	0.19
Luchun	0	–	238,010	0	0
Jinping	0	–	333,214	0	0
Hekou	1	–	1,107,618	0.01	0
Maguan	2	–	406,359	0.05	0
Malipo	–	–	313,477	0	0
Funing	–	–	452,800	0	0
Total	475	49			

2.4 Information 4: Preventing Malaria from Reintroduction

2.4.1 Objective

By the end of this part, learners should be able to know how to prevent malaria reintroduction, especially at border areas?

2.4.2 Goal and Strategy

Malaria transmission was finally and fully interrupted in 2016. The goal of phase 2017–2020 is to prevent malaria from reintroduction, continuously maintain malaria-free status, and pass the national certification of malaria elimination. Yunnan set up its goal of no introduced case， in spite of that the incidence of introduced cases does not influence the certification of malaria free.

According to WHO guidelines, the strategy includes proactive and reactive approaches and set up the following objectives:

1. Early detection and notification of all malaria cases and prompt diagnosis and treatment.
2. Assessment of possibility and potential causes of the reintroduction of malaria transmission.
3. Immediate action in the event of renewed local malaria transmission.
4. Determination of the risk of malaria reintroduction on the basis of and regular monitoring of receptivity and vulnerability of the area.

Yunnan Health and Family Planning Commission (YHFPC) distributed the notification on strengthening malaria surveillance for malaria elimination. The notification emphasized the strategy of universal coverage of malaria case surveillance. The strategy made clear the responsibility in malaria case surveillance to strengthen the health facility-based surveillance of malaria cases, and the county CDC-centered rapid response to any malaria cues to prevent malaria from reintroduction across Yunnan. Other health facilities that do not perform laboratory diagnosis such as private clinics and drug outlets are required to refer febrile patients with suspected malaria to the hospital and the county CDC where perform laboratory test (microscopy or RDTs) for detecting malaria. The rapid response of the county CDC should continuously follow the national "1-3-7" approach (YHFPC 2018a). To ensure certification of malaria-free, cross-border collaboration was continuously an important strategy to reduce the imported malaria.

To more effectively and pricisely prevent reintroduction of malaria, the YHFPC issued "The Protocol of Malaria Elimination Action Plan in Border High-Risk Areas of Yunnan Province" to identify the high-risk border villages where there were indigenous malaria cases during 2015–2016, and that are within a 2-km distance of malaria-endemic communities in neighboring countries. In 2018, a total of

16 natural villages were identified as high-risk border villages, as shown in Table 2.2, along with the detected malaria cases and their categories in 25 border counties (Table 2.3) (CNHC 2021).

Table 2.2 High-risk villages in 25 border counties in 2018

No.	Village name (high-risk village)	Located township	Located county (Type A)
1	Daoshui village 4	Nansan	Zhenkang
2	Yakou village	Mengdui	
3	Mengding Plantation division, Team 2	Mengding	Genma
4	Hanhong Mangbeng Village 1		
5	Manghai new market	Manghai	Mangshi
6	Xiabanlao village Longyaoshan	Banlao	Cangyuan
7	Nabang village qiaotou	Nabang	Yingjiang
8	Nabang village new national gate		
9	Nabang village Lisu natural village		
10	Nabang village Jingpo natural village		
11	Nabang village Kaya River		
12	Nabang village Laban port		
13	Street village vegetable team		
14	Daolong village		
15	Caobajie Dongpengyang	Kachang	
16	Longpen village	Taiping	

Table 2.3 Malaria cases detected and categories in 25 border counties, Yunnan 2017–2020

	2017	2018	2019	2020	Total
Total	264	169	149	137	719
Plasmodium spp					
P. falciparum	11	10	2	2	25
P. vivax	251	155	147	133	686
P. malariae	0	1	0	0	1
P. ovale	0	0	0	2	2
Mixed *(Pf + Pv)*	2	3	0	0	5
Location infected					
Indigenous cases	0	0	0	0	0
Imported cases	264	169	149	137	719
Counties					0
Tenchong	28	18	22	23	91
Longling	5	5		1	11
Jiangcheng	0	0	0	0	0
Menglian	0	1	0	0	1
Lancang	0	0	0	0	0
Ximeng	0	0	0	0	0
Zhenkang	0	1	0	0	1
Gengma	2	2	3	2	9
Cangyuan	3	1	5	8	17

(Continued)

Table 2.3 (Continued)

	2017	2018	2019	2020	Total
Jinping	1	2	1	2	6
Luchun	0	0	0	0	0
Hekou	0	0	0	0	0
Malipo	0	0	0	0	0
Maguan	0	1	0	0	1
Funing	0	1	0	0	1
Jinghong	0	1	0	0	1
Menghai	0	1	1	0	2
Mengla	1	1	0	0	2
Ruili	15	12	8	3	38
Mangshi	13	8	13	7	41
Yingjiang	179	106	92	75	452
Longchuan	17	8	4	16	45
Lushui	0	0	0	0	0
Fugong	0	0	0	0	0
Gongshan	0	0	0	0	0

2.4.3 Exercise

Question and Answer

7. How to face the remaining challenges of prevention of reintroduction (POR) for malaria in your own country?

(As an opening question)

Recommended time:

- 20 min

Refer to the information provided below and, in combination with the situation in your country, set up strategies to prevent malaria reintroduction.

Reference answer:

1. Establish and implement an efficient malaria surveillance system.
2. Maintain the budget for POR at least at the same level as before elimination.
3. Provide ongoing staff education/training programs for diagnosis, treatment, and vigilance for general health service personnel.
4. Ensure that training refreshers for diagnosis and treatment of malaria are regularly provided.
5. Establish or maintain malaria prevention services targeting the country/region/sub-region based on the epidemiological data sources (YHFPC 2018b).
6. Collaborating with entomologists and epidemiologists, particularly on activities targeting malaria vectors, to develop a national malaria prevention plan is also crucial (YHFPC 2018b).

In addition, general health services authorities are responsibile for detecting all suspected local and migrant malaria cases, notifying such cases and conducting epidemiological investigations, and administration of medication to each patient.

2.5 Information 5: The 3+1 Strategy Developed and Applied to Prevent Malaria from Reintroduction

Yunnan has been certified malaria-free nationally. However, it is still facing the problem of introduced malaria along its "'border seriously due to its special location and ecology." The national requirement is to prevent reestablishment of malaria transmission (YHFPC 2018b). Yunnan's long-term goal is to prevent malaria from reintroduction that is more ambitious than the national requirement. In order to effectively prevent reintroduction in border areas, Yunnan has formulated the "3 + 1″ strategy for border malaria elimination and cooperation, based on the experiences and lessons learned from border malaria control and elimination developed in 2019.

Border-spill malaria described in this case study is an imported malaria carried by infected anophelines who fly over the boundary from neighboring endemic areas and reintroduce malaria along the border areas of China. The border-spill malaria is related to the distance traveled by female anopheline mosquitoes. Experiments of 291 anopheline mosquito mark-release-recapture (MMRR) in 143 localities around the world estimated that the mean distance traveled (MDT) by female anophelines does not exceed 2.5 km (Guerra et al. 2014; Xu et al. 2021b).

Strategy 1 Intensive interventions are carried out within 2.5 km-wide perimeter along the border to prevent border-spill malaria.

The area within 2.5 km of the international border is the travel transmission radius of anopheline mosquitoes. Comprehensive interventions should include (1) passive and proactive case detection, (2) intensive surveillance of vectors, (3) vector control based on the data of surveillance, and (4) preventative treatment with antimalarial drugs based on the data of efficacy surveillance (Xu et al. 2021b).

Note: Operational research could be conducted on the knowledge, awareness, and practices of patients, as well as those of public and private health-care providers.

2.5.1 Exercise

Question and Answer
8. Does the border-spill malaria certainly happen within 2.5 km-wide perimeter? Why?
Reference answer:

- Not at all, the incidence of the border-spill malaria depends on the degree of endemicity in the border areas of neighboring countries, vector density and capacity, and malaria cross-border transmission intensity. The border-spill malaria may not or less happen when the malaria endemicity and vector density is very low in the border areas of neighboring countries.

Recommended time:

- 5–6 min

Strategy 2 Community based on migrants and travelers in frontier townships are carried out malaria detection and screening.

Unauthorized travelers often cross-border and appear in frontier townships. Strengthening the maintenance of malaria surveillance should include (1) in the township hospitals carry out passive malaria detection; (2) seeking assistance from village leaders and health workers, monitoring cross-border travelers, and referring febrile patients to the township hospitals; and (3) the CDC in the county maintains regular proactive case detection (Xu et al. 2021b).

2.5.2 Exercise

Question and Answer
9. Why should intensified malaria surveillance be maintained in a frontier township?
Reference answer:
According to China's administrative system, townships belong to the second bottom of six levels (e.g., national, provincial, prefecture, county, township, and village). The frontier townships mean along the international boundary townships. During the process of border malaria elimination, the frontier townships are facing following challenges:

1. Individuals who enter China without permission often appear in townships or towns along the international boundary (frontier townships). The median population of a frontier township is around 15,000 people.
2. In border areas, most of them are no natural or artificial barriers except for formal ports of entry and exit.

3. People of the same ethnic groups live on both sides of the border, some of whom are relatives or close friends.
4. In most border areas, the local residents walk freely across the border.
5. Passengers without entry permits into China include illegal immigrants, traders, visitors of relatives and friends, etc.
6. These passengers are at a high risk of carrying malaria infections, making it easy for malaria to be reintroduced and even reestablished in border areas of China.

Recommended discussion time:

- 10 min

Strategy 3 Carry out malaria surveillance throughout the province to detect malaria cues.

Passive detection should be integrated into the normal health services. Health services personnel should remain vigilant, ensure universal coverage of malaria detection and respond quickly to any malaria cues.

2.5.3 Exercise

Question and Answer

10. How to discover any suspected malaria cues? What is the key to find any malaria cases?

(As an opening question)

Reference answer:

In order to discover any suspected malaria cues, universal coverage of malaria surveillance, with the reduction of parasite reservoir, full surveillance has instituted. Its purpose is to discover evidence of sustained or recovered transmission, detect imported cases as early as possible, and provide a rapid and sufficient response. The individual functions of surveillance unit are as follows:

1. To detect all suspected malaria cases (including active and passive case detection).
2. Effectively treat all positive cases.
3. To carry out case investigation and genotyping of indigenous parasite isolates.
4. To carry out the epidemiological investigation of foci to determine their origin, extent, and classification.

5. To carry out parasitological surveys including active case detection.
6. To carry out entomological surveys.
7. To conduct meteorological monitoring.
8. Vector control and drug treatment are major remedial actions to further eliminate foci.
9. To promote and maintain community awareness and follow-up actions.
10. To enhance political mobilization to support continuous funding and investment.

In order to achieve 100% detection and notification of cases, it is necessary to involve the public, patients, and local authorities. The key to finding malaria cases, and thus to prevent it spreading, is maintaining the vigilance of health personnel toward malaria.

Strategy +1 To strengthen collaborative support with neighboring countries.

According to the agreement between the two countries, a comprehensive integrated control strategy should be carried out to reduce burden of malaria in both countries. Clear attention should be paid to border areas between neighboring countries (Xu et al. 2021b).

2.5.4 *Exercise*

Question and Answer
11. How to make sure effective cooperation with neighboring countries to carry out intervention activities smoothly?

(As an opening question)
Recommended time:

- 10 min

Reference answer:
Key points of answers include:

1. Obtain the commitment of bilateral governments to cooperate.
2. To establish an agreed framework and authorize corresponding local government agencies and civil society organization to carry out mutually beneficial activities. For example, Yunnan border area between China and Myanmar signed the Cross-Border Malaria Prevention and Control Agreement on June 7, 2005. With the support of the international collaboration department, China National Health Commission (the former Ministry of Health) fully cooperates/integrates with the private health sec-

tor. Yunnan has carried out "The joint malaria control project along China–Myanmar Border" since 2005.

12. How to guide and promote case management for malaria elimination, including diagnosis and the use of antimalarial drugs?

(As an opening question)

Recommended time:

- 20 min

Reference answer:

Key points of answers include:

We should encourage participants to think of ideas for operational research on issues of parasitological diagnosis and antimalarial drug use, as well as the evaluation of possible intervention measures.

1. The participation of the private sector in formative studies on managing malaria cases should be assessed, such as by using surrogate patients or through substantive studies like controlled trials, for example, by use of an incentive scheme.
2. The compliance of the 14-day primaquine regimen could be studied by observing the treatment outcomes of *vivax* malaria patients who self-administer the medication, compared to those receive treatment from health-care workers on a daily basis. Patients could seek medical attention at home and are required to present their primaquine package after, for example, 12 days.
3. What is the importance of eliminating *Plasmodium vivax* in Africa?
4. Need to conduct more research on the side effects of primaquine in different populations, as well as the newly proposed high-dose of primaquine for treatment of *Plasmodium vivax*.
5. New diagnostic tests for available glucose-6-phosphate dehydrogenase (G6PD) deficiency should be introduced, as the unclear G6PD activity level of patient limits the potential use of primaquine as radical treatment of *vivax* malaria and *ovals* malaria.
6. Clinical trials can be conducted, such as studying the knowledge, awareness, and practices of patients as well as public and private health-care providers.
7. Field studies to compare the cost-effectiveness of IRS and LLINs.
8. To determine the diagnostics methods used by the private sector and their sensitivity and specificity through some applied researches.

Acknowledgments This work was supported by the Bill & Melinda Gates Foundation (No. INV-018913).

References

China National Health Commission (2021) The governance of preventing re-establishment of malaria transmission. China National Health Commission, Beijing. Accessed 30 January 2019 (in Chinese)

Guerra AC, Reiner JRR, Perkins TA, Lindsay SW, Midega JT, Brady O et al (2014) A global assembly of adult female mosquito mark-release-recapture data to inform the control of mosquito-borne pathogens. Parasit Vectors 7:276

Ma J, Yang G, Shi X (2006) Disease surveillance based information technology platform in China [in Chinese]. Ji Bing Jian Ce 21:1–3

Xu JW, Liu H (1997) Border malaria in Yunnan, China. Southeast Asian J Trop Med Public Health 28:456

Xu JW, Lee R, Li XH, Hui L (2021a) Transition of radical, preventive and presumptive treatment regimens for malaria in China: a systematic review. Malar J 20:10

Xu JW, Lin ZR, Zhou YW et al (2021b) Intensive surveillance, rapid response and border collaboration for malaria elimination: China Yunnan's "3+1"strategy. Malar J 20:396

Yang W, Li Z, Lan Y (2011) A nationwide web-based automated system for outbreak early detection and rapid response in China. WPSAR, World Health Organization Regional Office for the Western Pacific, Manila, p 2

Yunna Health and Family Planning Commission (2018a) The notification on further standardizing malaria elimination work and process. Yunnan Health and Family Planning Commission, Kunming. Accessed 27 Feb 2019 (in Chinese)

Yunnan Health and Family Planning Commission (2018b) The protocol of malaria elimination action plan in border high risk areas of Yunnan Province. Yunnan Health and Family Planning Commission, Kunming. Accessed 16 July 2019 (in Chinese)

Chapter 3
The Three-Layer Strategy (TLS) Promoted Malaria Elimination Among Forest-Goers in Hainan Island

Yu-Chun Li, Guang-Ze Wang, Wen Zeng, Xiao-Min Huang, Feng Meng, Ding-Wei Sun, Shuai Wang, and Dan Wang

Theme
The three-layer strategy for interruption of malaria transmission.

Target Audience
Public health workers, government officials, and researchers involved in malaria control or elimination.

Learning Objectives
Upon finishing this case study, participants should be able to:

1. Comprehend the natural environment, vectors, and high-risk groups associated with the malaria epidemic in Hainan Island.
2. Recognize the malaria control strategies for individuals visiting forests.
3. Acquire proficiency in implementing malaria epidemic control measures for forest visitors during the elimination phase.

Overview
Hainan Island, located in the southernmost tropical region of China, has historically faced significant malaria outbreaks mainly due to *Plasmodium falciparum* and *P. vivax*. (Xia et al. 2014). Through nearly seven decades of persistent efforts, malaria has gradually been eliminated in Hainan Island. The island's tropical monsoon and marine climates, featuring diverse terrains like mountains, hills, plateaus, and plains, create perfect breeding environments for malaria-carrying vectors such as *Anopheles dirus* and *An. minimus*. Before its elimination, malaria cases in Hainan Island were mainly concentrated in the southwestern areas of Hainan Island. Since the 1990s, individuals venturing into forests have been identified as a high-risk

Y.-C. Li · G.-Z. Wang · W. Zeng · X.-M. Huang · F. Meng · D.-W. Sun · S. Wang
D. Wang (✉)
Hainan Provincial Center for Disease Control and Prevention,
Haikou, Hainan, People's Republic of China

X.-N. Zhou, J.-H. Yin (eds.), *Malaria Control and Elimination in China*,
https://doi.org/10.1007/978-981-97-8719-7_3

group for malaria transmission, emphasizing the need to target this demographic in Hainan's malaria control strategies.

Forest-goers, including both locals and migrants who stay overnight in the mountains for activities like harvesting and planting, significantly contribute to the dynamics of malaria transmission. This case study seeks to emphasize the importance of surveillance and response actions aimed at forest-goers to disrupt malaria transmission in the mountainous regions of Sanya City, Hainan Province. The three-layer strategy (TLS) applied in this study has shown to be an efficient method in addressing localized malaria outbreaks during the elimination phase, providing valuable insights that can benefit similar regions encountering similar obstacles.

3.1 Part 1. General Information

3.1.1 Nature and Geographic Information of Hainan Island

Hainan Island, located at the southernmost tip of China, is bordered by the Qiongzhou Strait to the north, the Beibuwan Gulf to the west, the South China Sea and Taiwan Province to the east, and the Philippines, Brunei, and Malaysia to the southeast and south in the South China Sea (Fig. 3.1). Resembling a large oval pear from northeast to southwest, Hainan Island covers a total area of 33,900 km^2, ranking as the second largest island in China after Taiwan Island. The island experiences a tropical monsoon climate with extended summers and no winters, featuring an average annual temperature ranging from 22 °C to 27 °C and an average annual precipitation of 1639 mm.

The central region of Hainan Island is marked by prominent elevations, including the core mountains of Wuzhishan, Yingge, and Bawangling, which gradually taper toward the periphery. Wuzhishan Mountain, centrally positioned, showcases a primary peak rising to 1867.1 m above sea level, claiming the title of the island's highest summit. Northwest of Wuzhishan Mountain lies Yingge Mountain, with its main

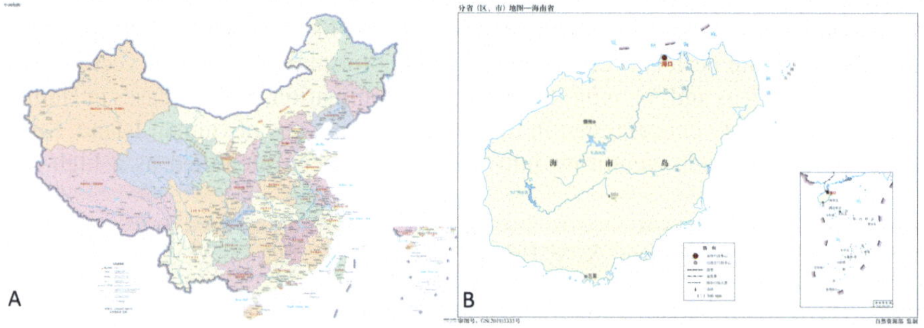

Fig. 3.1 Nature and geographic maps in Hainan, China. (**a**) Map of China (GS(2022)4316); (**b**) Map of Hainan (GS(2019)3333): 海南岛 (Hainan island); 海口市 (Haikou city); 三亚市 (Sanya city); 儋州市 (Danzhou city)

peak reaching 1811.6 m. In the island's western expanse sits Bawang Mountain, featuring a principal peak at 1560 m. Other mountains on Hainan Island vary between 500 and 800 m, forming a landscape of hills and low valleys. The majority of rivers originate from the central mountainous regions, forming a network of waterways that include the Nandu River, Changhua River, and Wanquan River. While natural lakes and artificial various reservoirs are scarce on Hainan Island such as Songtao, Niululing, Daguangba, and Nanli Lake are scattered across the area.

3.1.2 General Information on Malaria and Vectors in Hainan Province

Tropical plants such as coconuts, areca nuts, and rubber trees thrive in the optimal tropical monsoon and marine climate of Hainan Province, providing a conducive environment for the breeding of major malaria vectors, including *An. dirus* and *An. minimus* (Wei et al. 2007). Malaria outbreaks have been a recurring issue on Hainan Island although the malaria annual incidence has been kept at low level after 2000 due to intensive control program. Since 2010, there have been consistent reports of indigenous cases of *P. falciparum* and *P. vivax* infections on the island (Yin et al. 2014).

Sanya City, located at the southern tip of Hainan Island, falls within the tropical climate zone influenced by the nearby Pacific Ocean. The city experiences an annual average temperature of 25.7 °C. Sanya was historically a primary endemic area for malaria in Hainan Province, with both *P. vivax* and *P. falciparum* strains prevalent. The region's geographical characteristics create an ideal tropical climate that supports year-round reproduction of malaria vectors. *An. minimus* is recognized as a significant vector found in the mountainous areas of Sanya, alongside *An. sinensis* (Wei et al. 2007).

Gaofeng Township, situated on the outskirts of Sanya City and bordered by Baoting County, Ledong County, and Wuzhishan City, features high mountains, dense forests, and abundant natural resources. This environment provides an ideal breeding ground for mosquitoes, increasing the risk of malaria transmission among the local population. Local residents, known as forest-goers, who live in and spend nights in the hills or mountains, are particularly susceptible to malaria infections and often suffer from the disease. In recent years, these forest-goers have been engaging in activities such as collecting red vine fruit and honey, driven by the high market value of these products from March to December annually.

Question and Answer

1. What are your thoughts on the geographic and natural characteristics of Hainan Island?

(As an opening question to raise interest)

Reference answer 1:

- Hainan Island, is shaped like a snow pear and stands as China's second-largest island. Positioned at the northern edge of tropical islands, Hainan Island boasts a tropical monsoon climate without a distinct winter season.

The island maintains an average annual temperature ranging from 22 °C to 27 °C and receives an average annual precipitation of 1639 mm. It experiences clearly defined rainy and dry seasons. The central region of Hainan Island showcases diverse terrain, with the Nandu River, Changhua River, and Wanquan River meandering through the area, along with several lakes.
Recommended discussion time:

- 5 min

2. Can you introduce the geographical and natural environment of your country or region?
Reference answer 2:

- For example, in Tanzania, the situation is…
Recommended discussion time:

- 10 min

3. How many major vectors of malaria are found in Hainan Island? Remember one or more?
Reference answer 3:

- *Anopheles dirus, Anopheles mininus, Anopheles sinensis*
Recommended discussion time:

- 3 min

3.1.3 History of Malaria Surveillance in Sanya City and Hainan Province

Malaria-endemic areas in Hainan Province have been grappling with infections of *P. falciparum* and *P. vivax*. Since 1954, an annual parasite survey of local residents (PSLR) has been conducted in Hainan Island as part of active case detection (ACD). Before 1964, PSLR data indicated an average of 10 cases (CI: 2–42) of *P. malariae* infections confirmed annually on Hainan Island (Yin et al. 2014).

In Sanya City, PSLR initiatives have been ongoing since 1959, focusing mainly on detecting cases of *P. falciparum* and *P. vivax* infections. However, it was not until 2015 that cases of *P. malariae* were identified. During the malaria elimination program from 2011 to 2018, Sanya City reported eight locally acquired cases and six imported cases. Indigenous cases of *P. vivax* infection were recorded in 2011, with no cases reported between 2012 and 2014. In 2015, six indigenous cases of *P. malariae* infection were identified, while no cases were reported in 2017 (Figs. 3.2 and 3.3).

Question and Answer
4. Which kinds of malaria parasites were presented in Hainan Island and in Sanya City, respectively?

Reference answer 4:

- Historically, Hainan Island was affected by three malaria species: *P. falciparum*, *P. vivax*, and *P. malariae*. However, case infected with *P. malariae* has not been found in Sanya after 1964, while cases of *P. falciparum* and *P. vivax* were reported as indigenous infections prior to elimination efforts. Recommended discussion time:
- 5 min

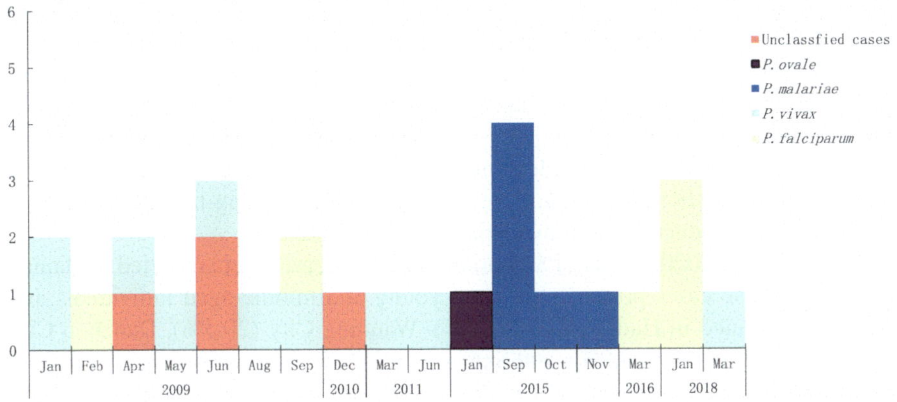

Fig. 3.2 Distribution of malaria cases by different species in four seasons in Sanya City, Hainan Province

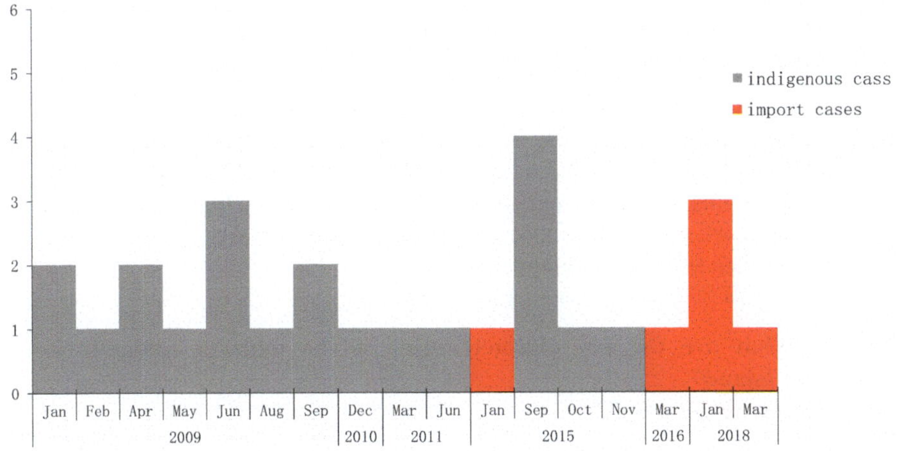

Fig. 3.3 Distribution of indigenous and imported malaria cases in four seasons from 2009 to 2018 in Sanya City, Hainan Province

3.1.4 High-Risk Group for Malaria Transmission in Hainan Province

Forest-goers, referring to individuals who spend nights in the mountains for activities like harvesting and planting, consist of both local residents and temporary migrants (Xia et al. 2014). In 2002, the infection rate among forest-goers stood at 30.9% (95 out of 307 individuals), more than double that of residents who did not venture into the forests (15.2%). Factors contributing to malaria occurrence among forest-goers include the duration of their mountain stays, adherence to antimalarial treatment, acceptance of malaria prevention campaigns, and the use of mosquito control measures (Li et al. 2022a, b).

Since the 1990s, Hainan Province has actively engaged in malaria control and pre-elimination endeavors. A targeted approach to prevent and manage malaria among forest-goers has been reinforced through support from a project funded by the Global Fund Against HIV/AIDS, Tuberculosis, and Malaria (GFATM) since 2003. This strategy emphasizes effectively performing mass drug administration (MDA) to patients and their close contacts (family members or colleagues or neighbors), conducting precise epidemiological investigations, promptly monitoring vector populations, and swiftly implementing vector control measures such as indoor residual spraying (IRS), insecticide-treated nets (ITNs), or long-lasting insecticidal nets (LLINs) to reduce malaria incidence (Li et al. 2022a, b).

From 2011 to 2020, a total of 88 imported malaria cases were reported in Hainan Province. These cases primarily affected young and middle-aged individuals and were concentrated in Haikou City (43.2%), Wanning City (20.5%), Danzhou City (9.1%), Dongfang City (8.0%), and Sanya City (6.8%). The imported cases mainly originated from 23 countries across three continents, including Africa (68 cases, 77.27%), Asia (19 cases, 21.59%), and Oceania (1 case, 1.14%) (Li et al. 2022a, b).

Question and Answer

5. Who are the main high-risk groups in Hainan Island?

Reference answer 5:

- Prior to malaria elimination, indigenous cases in Hainan Island predominantly affected forest-goers, who constituted the primary high-risk population. However, during the malaria elimination phase, the importance of imported malaria cases from abroad, also identified as a high-risk group in recent years, must not be underestimated in Hainan Island.
  Recommended discussion time:
- 2 min

6. What are the key characteristics of the malaria epidemic in Hainan Island?

Reference answer 6:

- Forest-goers have been identified as a high-risk population for malaria transmission in Hainan Island since the 1990s. Control measures, includ-

ing MDA, epidemiological investigations, and vector control, targeting forest-goers have been tailored and effectively implemented to reduce malaria incidence in Hainan Island. Before elimination, there were predominantly *P. vivax* and *P. falciparum* infections as indigenous cases. In recent years, some imported malaria cases from abroad have been observed.
Recommended discussion time:

- 2 min

7. Does your country have endemic malaria on an island similar to Hainan Island?

What is the specific situation, and how can interventions target malaria vectors and high-risk groups? (as an opening question to generate interest)

Reference answer 7:

- For instance, in Tanzania, the situation was...
  Recommended discussion time:
- 10 min

3.2 Part 2. An Outbreak of Malaria

On September 7, 2015, a man visited the Sanya Hospital of Agricultural Reclamation for outpatient care, presenting symptoms of chills, fever, headache, and limb weakness (Lin et al. 2016). The next day, malaria parasites were identified in blood smear slides through microscopy examination. These slides were then sent to the Sanya City and Hainan Center for Disease Control and Prevention (CDC) for confirmation. Ultimately, on September 14, he received a diagnosis of *P. malariae* infection based on laboratory tests. Epidemiological investigation revealed that he resided in Hongqi village, Baolong village committee, Gaofeng Township, Tianya district, Sanya City. His symptoms first appeared in June, and he sought medical help from various village doctors and hospitals before finally receiving a diagnosis on September 7 at the Sanya Hospital of Agricultural Reclamation. This case marked the initial instance or index case of *P. malariae* infections in Gaofeng Township, Sanya City.

Question and Answer

8. What are the key components of the 1-3-7 surveillance and response approach?

Reference answer 8:

- Based on the malaria elimination strategy of "clear foci, following clues," the 1-3-7 surveillance and response approach has been in place in China since 2012 (Cao et al. 2014). It involves reporting cases within 1 day, investigating cases within 3 days, and investigating and taking action on transmission foci within 7 days. Response measures for foci include mass drug administration (MDA), vector surveillance, indoor residual spraying (IRS), and distributing insecticide-treated nets (ITNs) or long-lasting insecticidal nets (LLINs).

Recommended discussion time:

- 2 min

9. As a staff member in a malaria control program, what steps should you take when a malaria case is reported from a hospital?

Reference answer 9:

To validate the index case, it is crucial to review epidemiological records, clinical symptoms, and laboratory test results.

- If the case is determined to be false, the alarm should be promptly dismissed.
- If the case is confirmed, it is important to identify the specific vectors responsible for transmission, conduct a comprehensive epidemiological investigation, and implement targeted interventions to address and eliminate the transmission focus.

Recommended discussion time:

- 3 min

10. What steps should the public health department take after confirming an index case of malaria?

Reference answer 10:

The following steps should be taken after confirming an index case of malaria:

- Validate the laboratory findings from the hospital report with CDC technicians to confirm the presence of malaria parasites in the blood smear slides and determine the species through both slides and nucleic acid analysis.
- Consult with clinicians regarding the patient's clinical evidence, utilizing information such as clinical laboratory results, hospital observations, symptom onset, to develop a treatment plan and implement mosquito control measures in the hospital ward.
- Gather epidemiological investigation data, including personal details, family size, recent travel history, blood transfusions, coworker interactions, overnight stays in forests, etc.
- Ensure the accuracy of the collected information through multiple inquiries and verification processes. If needed, involve public security or other relevant departments to track down necessary details.

Recommended discussion time:

- 3 min

11. Which actions should be taken to prevent the spread of this epidemic after foci investigation finished with accurate information?

Reference answer 11:

The following actions should be taken to prevent the spread of this epidemic after foci investigation finished with accurate information:

- Mobilize a diverse team of professionals to engage in epidemic management, comprising laboratory personnel, epidemiologists, vector surveillance experts, and logistical support staffs.
- Develop comprehensive plans, assign specific tasks and responsibilities, and ensure that all necessary materials are available.
- Gather historical data on malaria prevalence, including information on vectors, over the past decade.
- Identify and categorize the focal point as an active epidemic site.
- Investigate potential contacts based on clues from the index case's epidemiological profile, conduct blood smear collection for potential contacts.
- Interview and examine family members, neighbors, and colleagues of the index case to gather personal and health information and collect blood samples.
- Conduct vector surveys and implement indoor residual spraying measures in the vicinity of the foci.
- Compile census data from the community or village for future screening using blood slides.

These measures align with the tailored implementation of the 1-3-7 approach in Hainan island.

Recommended discussion time:

- 5 min

3.3 Part 3. Case Screening and Epidemiological Investigation

Guided by the index case (Case 1), the 1-3-7 surveillance and response strategy was implemented in the community area where the index case lives (Tables 3.1 and 3.2). Subsequently, three cases of *P. malariae* malaria (Case 2, Case 3, and Case 4) were detected from September 15 to September 19. Additionally, on October 15, a patient (Case 5) with a fever actively sought medical care at the township-level hospital and was subsequently diagnosed with a *P. malariae* infection (Lin et al. 2016).

Table 3.1 The Surveillance Date on Malaria Prevalence Collected from 2004 to 2014 in Sanya City[a]

	Febrile patients[b]							Non- febrile patients			
				Species						Species	
Year	No. slides	No. positive	Positive ratio (%)	*Pv*	*Pf*	mix	No. slides	No. positive	Ratio (%)	*Pv*	*Pf*
2004	16,994	1116	6.57	743	368	5	1972	8	0.41	3	5
2005	15,969	267	1.67	215	50	2	2202	20	0.91	20	0
2006	15,053	122	0.81	106	16	0	1504	14	0.93	11	3
2007	25,846	108	0.42	65	42	1	529	1	0.19	0	1
2008	15,709	44	0.28	39	5	0	981	1	0.1	1	0
2009	19,519	6	0.03	4	2	0	1141	1	0.09	1	0
2010	19,518	0	0	0	0	0	520	0	0	0	0
2011	14,516	2	0.01	2	0	0	852	0	0	0	0
2012[c]	12,071	0	0	0	0	0	200	0	0	0	0
2013	11,884	0	0	0	0	0	553	0	0	0	0
2014	11,665	0	0	0	0	0	250	0	0	0	0
合计Total	227,790	3490	20.85	2436	1040	14	19,756	122	5.62	95	27

[a]From the report of elimination malaria in Sanya

[b]From some surveillance archives and published articles, the positive ratio of malaria infection in febrile patients in Sanya have been declined from 6.5% to 0. The ratio of residents with malaria infection have been declined from 0.91% to 0. From 2012 to 2014, there were no reports of indigenous malaria cases and no imported malaria cases in Sanya for three consecutive years. At the same time, the results of residents' malaria in survey showed that there were no malaria carriers

[c]The last indigenous malaria case of *P. vivax* in Hainan island was reported in 2012 in Sanya

Table 3.2 Vector information in Sanya City from 2000 to 2014

Years	No. sites	Total no.	*An. minus*	*An. dirus*	Others[a]
2004	14	1077	23	0	1054
2005	14	1372	22	0	1350
2006	2	510	5	0	505
2007	1	172	0	0	172
2008	1	724	3	0	721
2009	1	444	0	0	444
2010	3	572	0	0	572
2011	1	1242	2	0	1240
2012	1	1618	0	0	1618
2013	3	1248	0	0	1248
2014	1	1170	0	0	1170

[a]This data includes the number of *An. sinensis*

Question and Answer

12. Faced with the three newly identified cases, what steps should be taken next?

Reference answer 12:

- Conduct a detailed analysis of demographic characteristics, including time, regional, and population distributions, and epidemiological characteristics such as treatment patterns, pre-diagnosis activities, and clinical features.

  Recommended discussion time:

- 2 min

13. What is the next step following the appearance of case 5 in the outpatient setting?

Reference answer 13:

- Reapply the 1–3-7 approach toolkit for case 5 and identify two coworkers. However, two individuals tested negative for malaria upon blood slide examination.

  Recommended discussion time:

- 2 min

After the detection of five malaria cases through the implementation of the 1-3-7 surveillance and response approach, an additional case of *P. malariae* infection (Case 6) was identified during active case detection at the local hospital on November 26. Epidemiological investigations revealed that all five initial cases (Case 1, Case 2, Case 3, Case 4, Case 5) experienced fever after overnight stays in the mountainous regions and were categorized as forest-goers. However, Case 6 solely had a fever without any history of being a forest-goer (Table 3.3).

Table 3.3 History records of six cases found in Gaofeng Township of Sanya City

Cases	Species of parasite	Resident village	Date diagnosed	Forest-goer	Way of surveillance
Case 1	*Plasmodium malariae*	Baolong Village, Gaofeng Township, Sanya City	September 14, 2015	Yes	Passive case detection
Case 2	*Plasmodium malariae*	Lixin Village, Gaofeng Township, Sanya City	September 15, 2015	Yes	Active case detection
Case 3	*Plasmodium malariae*	Lixin Village, Gaofeng Township, Sanya City	Sept 17, 2015	Yes	Active case detection
Case 4	*Plasmodium malariae*	Lixin Village, Gaofeng Township, Sanya City	September 19 2015	Yes	Active case detection
Case 5	*Plasmodium malariae*	Zhanan Village, Gaofeng Township, Sanya City	October 17, 2015	Yes	Passive case detection
Case 6	*Plasmodium malariae*	Lixin Village, Gaofeng Township, Sanya City	November 26, 2015	No	Active case detection

The first five cases engaged in activities like harvesting bodhi fruit (*Daemonoropus margaritae* Becc var. *palawanica*) or collecting honey in the mountains year-round. Case 1, who was part of a group with Cases 2, 3, and 4, and Case 5, along with two others, went mountain climbing and spent the night gathering bodhi fruit. Conversely, Case 6 never stayed overnight in the mountains and remained within the villages. The onset of *P. malariae* infection in Cases 1 to 5 is attributed to their nights spent in the mountains. Additionally, a villager from Case 6 also contracted *P. malariae* infection in the same village where some malaria cases were reported (Fig. 3.4).

Question and Answer

14. Is there a chance that the 1-3-7 approach could be ineffective in the presence of potential transmission?

Reference answer 14:

- After implementing the 1-3-7 surveillance and response strategy, active case detection (ACD) was launched based on the information provided by case 1. The epidemiological profiles of three coworkers closely resembled that of case 1. However, the potential presence of other unconfirmed sources of infection or transmission in rural areas remains unconfirmed. While the 1-3-7 approach has shown efficacy for tracing imported malaria cases, the lack of systematic measures to prevent malaria local transmission has been noticeable since 2015.

  Recommended discussion time:

- 2 min

15. How should mass screening be organized and what factors need to be considered?

Reference answer 15:

The purpose of mass screening is to trace the origins of infection which help to stop the further spreading or transmission of malaria. So following factors need to be considered during implementation of mass screening (Zhou et al. 2015).

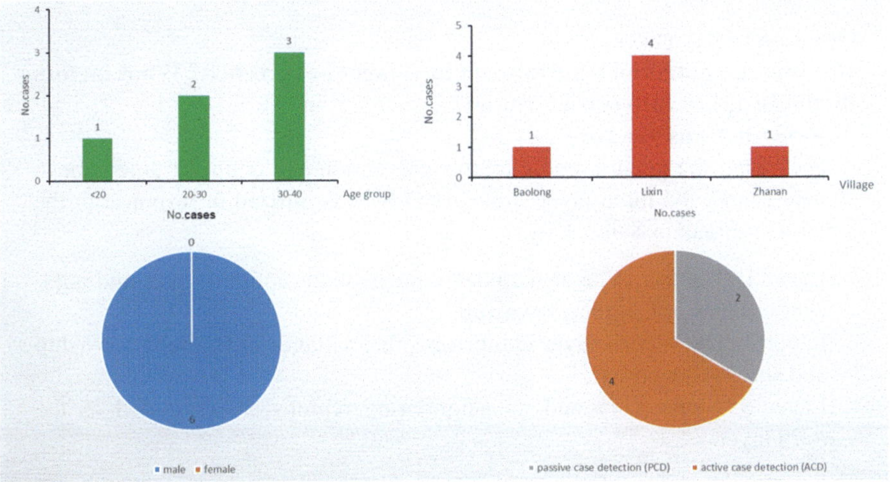

Fig. 3.4 Distribution of six *P. malariae* infections in outbreak foci of Sanyan City, Hainan island

- Gather basic information of local residents and compile lists.
- Provide training for public health workers and microscopists before conducting blood slide collection from residents, covering procedures like numbering, blood sampling, slide preparation, and staining.
- Inform villagers about the purpose and importance of the screening, ensuring informed consent before sampling.
- Schedule residents for sampling at specific times, guided by local community or village staff.
- Stain the collected blood samples and assign them to microscopists for malaria examination.

Recommended discussion time:

- 2 min

3.4 Part 4. Timely Response to the Outbreak

Immediately following the identification of Case 6, the potential for transmission cannot be overlooked. To mitigate this risk, it is crucial to screen the entire population in the outbreak-affected village and neighboring areas to pinpoint the potential source of infection.

As an island where less imported cases compared with that in mainland, the implementation of the three-layer strategy (TLS) was proposed and put into action, showcasing its cost-effectiveness, especially tailored for Hainan Island. The TLS also offers a more effective approach to solidify the gains made in the malaria elimination program.

Question and Answer

16. How can potential transmission in villages be screened? What factors should be taken into consideration?

Reference answer 16:

Following the malaria collaborative prevention and control framework in Hainan island, the three-layer strategy (TLS) was utilized in response to the malaria outbreak in Sanya City.

- Layer 1: The initial layer includes villages with reported cases and adjacent villages of Gaofeng township.
- Layer 2: The second layer comprises other villages in Gaofeng township and surrounding areas.
- Layer 3: Sanya City and its neighboring regions are classified as the third layer.

Key factors to consider:

- Geographical distribution of malaria cases
- Demographics of the population
- Past involvement in malaria control initiatives
- Operational requirements of the 1-3-7 strategy

Recommended discussion time:

- 2 min

17. What measures are implemented in each layer to prevent malaria transmission? How can these measures be designed in detail?

Reference answer 17:

- The measures involves blood slide and nucleic acid screening for all residents in the first layer.
- The measures includes blood slide screening for forest-goers and passive monitoring in hospitals in the second layer.
- The measures features passive monitoring in hospitals and health education for forest-goers in the third layer.

Recommended discussion time:

- 2 min

18. How can the planned prevention and control measures be implemented across the three layers effectively?

Reference answer 18:

Following actions could be taken to address effectively on implementation of TLS.

- Develop unified documentation, provide training, and delegate responsibilities through government channels with collaboration from multiple sectors.

- Execute actions in alignment with document guidelines and local conditions.
- Monitor the quality of actions and ensure adherence to the scheduled progress.
- Reflect on lessons learned.

Recommended discussion time:

- 2 min

19. Given the significant advantages of TLS, what role do you envision it playing in outbreak control?

Reference answer 19:

- TLS was first employed during a malaria outbreak in Hainan island, focusing on passive case detection (PCD) and active case detection (ACD). The strategy included:
  - Identifying high-risk individuals, such as frequent forest visitors among local and nearby residents, for ACD in targeted villages and surrounding regions.
  - Screening forest-goers for malaria if they had recent fever symptoms, considering them at high risk.
  - Providing health education to forest-goers to enhance awareness of malaria risks, advising against overnight stays in mountainous areas during the period, and encouraging prompt medical attention if needed.
  - Conducting PCR testing on blood samples from the high-risk group and suspicious samples from other layers to ensure accuracy.
- Vector surveillance and control measures were also implemented, targeting *An. dirus* and *An. minimus* with bait traps and *An. sinensis* with lamps. Monthly surveillance activities were conducted throughout the year in Hainan island due to continuous malaria transmission, with specific vector control methods including:
  - Indoor residual spraying (IRS) for *An. sinensis* and *An. minimus*.
  - Distribution of long-lasting insecticide nets (LLINs) as the primary method to prevent *An. dirus* and *An. minimus* transmission.

Recommended discussion time:

- 5 min

3.5 Part 5. Sustaining the Surveillance and Response Approach

Following the implementation of TLS in response to the malaria outbreak in 2015, no indigenous malaria case has been reported in Hainan Province since 2016. In order to meet the target of eliminating malaria by 2020, Hainan Province implemented rigorous measures using the TLS strategy between 2016 and 2018. These measures encompassed preventive treatment, vector surveillance, malaria tracking, training sessions, and various other initiatives. The utilization of TLS through sustained surveillance and response approach has notably hastened the progress toward malaria elimination in Hainan Province.

Question and Answer

20. What factors should be considered for individuals taking preventive medication?

Reference answer 20:

Following factors need to be considered for individual medication.

- Give priority to residents and individuals frequenting forests for preventive medication, administering it to all residents in the first layer and forest-goers in the second layer.
- Customize treatments according to specific groups, with a particular emphasis on children and individuals with diabetes.
- Ensure that informed consent is obtained.
- Establish a plan for managing any adverse reactions.

Administer medication to high-risk groups for three consecutive years, resulting in zero reported cases or local infection in Hainan Province since 2016.

Recommended discussion time:

- 1 min

21. What specific measures can be taken to enhance malaria control in TLS?

Reference answer 21:

The following specific measures can be taken to enhance the quality of TLS:

- Administer medication to high-risk groups across different layers.
- Regularly monitor and control vectors.
- Provide ongoing training to maintain alertness and precision in identifying cases.

Recommended discussion time:

- 1 min

22. Despite the innovative combination of TLS and the 1-3-7 approach for the first time in malaria elimination program in Hainan island, there are still shortcomings and constraints. What are the limitations of this case study?

Reference answer 22:

The limitations of this case study can be reflected in the following two aspects:

- While TLS was first implemented in 2015, there have been no comparable application scenarios in China to assess the feasibility of TLS post-2015.

- The link between two transmission chains remains uncertain, necessitating a fresh perspective, even though at least two transmission chains have been identified through epidemiological investigations.

Recommended discussion time:

- 1 min

3.6 Part 6. Summary

In 2015, a total of six cases of *P. malariae* were reported in Sanya city. With the exception of the index case (Case 1), all other cases were swiftly reported within 24 h through the Integrated Disease Information and Response Management System (IDIRMS). Based on IDIRMS data, these six individuals had no history of international travel, or blood transfusions, leading to their classification as indigenous malaria cases caused by *P. malariae* infections. The affected individuals, all male farmers aged 19–40, belonged to the younger-middle age group. Among them, 16% (Case 1) received a malaria diagnosis at a county-level hospital, while 33% (cases 1 and 5) underwent treatment at higher-level health-care facilities such as township or county hospitals.

Microscopic examination and sequencing techniques were employed for case detection, occurring between September and November. Three cases were documented in September, one in October, and one was confirmed in November. The indigenous malaria cases were concentrated in 3 villages of Gaofeng Township, accounting for 100% of cases in Sanya city, Hainan island. While Case 1 and 5 were identified through passive case detection (PCD), the remaining four cases were discovered through active case detection (ACD) within their respective villages. Outpatient visit data revealed that all individuals seeking treatment for febrile cases were attended to at local village clinics.

Question and Answer

22. What factors attributed to the cause of this outbreak?

Reference answer 22:

Following factors have been identified as contributing to the outbreak:

- Surveillance system sensitivity: The lack of sensitivity in surveillance systems played a crucial role in this outbreak. With no reports of indigenous malaria cases in Sanya City for three consecutive years, the malaria control departments adjusted or reduced their monitoring efforts. This relaxation led to changes in the roles and positions of personnel involved in malaria control.
- Lack of awareness: A significant factor was the lack of antimalarial awareness, especially among patients with lower educational backgrounds who

lack health knowledge. Villagers displayed weak self-protection awareness, with a low utilization rate of mosquito nets, particularly during field operations in mountainous regions.

- Inadequate health education: The absence of suitable health education exacerbated the issue. Targeted publicity of malaria prevention and control knowledge did not align with the acceptance ability and participation consciousness of Li and Miao minority villagers.
- Resurgence of *P. malariae*: The resurgence of *P. malariae* raised concerns due to its long incubation period. Infected individuals may carry the parasite for life, potentially leading to malaria attacks even after 20 to 30 years without repeated febrile cases. The low infection density when *P. malariae* infects aging red blood cells increases the likelihood of it being overlooked or misdiagnosed.
- Misdiagnosis: Misdiagnosis, particularly mistaking *P. vivax* for *P. malariae*, has been a common issue. Misdiagnosed carriers of *P. malariae* pose a risk as they remain asymptomatic and harbor parasites.
- Zoonotic transmission: The potential zoonotic transmission of *P. knowlesi*, the fifth *Plasmodium* species capable of infecting humans, is also a concern. The discovery of cases with a history of overnight mountain visits suggests a possible link to macaques encountered during field operations in mountainous areas.

Recommended discussion time:

- 5 min

23. What potential source of infection is responsible for this outbreak?

Reference answer 23:

Analysis of the mosquito-borne malaria cases suggests three potential sources of infection: Possible 1 (P1) related to the extended incubation period of *P. malaria*, possible 2 (P2) involving transmission from imported infections and subsequent reintroduction, and possible 3 (P3) indicating transmission from animal hosts in forested areas. Which of these scenarios is the most plausible?

- Considering the epidemiological patterns observed in these cases, particularly the age demographics, the second scenario seems the most credible, with the third scenario also holding merit. The first scenario, on the other hand, is deemed highly improbable.
- Recent reports on *P. malariae* cases originating mainly from Guangdong Province and Shanghai municipality of China suggest that *P. malariae* might result in persistent infections due to its prolonged incubation period, regardless of whether patients display recurring fevers. These cases predominantly impact older age groups rather than the typical young-to-middle age groups, marking a significant difference in this outbreak.

- The theory of human-to-monkey transmission lacks substantial evidence due to the limited number of confirmed cases (currently only 5). Although forest-goers interacting with macaques have been noted since 2015, no subsequent cases have been reported in these regions. Nonetheless, the potential for macaques to carry *P. malariae* cannot be dismissed. All malaria parasites identified in this outbreak have been confirmed as *P. malariae* rather than *P. simium* that responsible for zoonotic transmissions among forest-goers in Brazil. Therefore, we could not support the credibility of P3.
- Sanya, a vibrant tourist destination with a diverse population of Chinese residents and foreign nationals, harbors *An. minimus*, the primary malaria vector in Hainan island. The current study suggests that human-to-mosquito-to-human transmission among forest-goers is the most probable mode of transmission.

Recommended discussion time:

- 3 min

3.7 Part 7. Look Forward to the Future

Hainan Province achieved national validation for malaria elimination in 2020, following the last reported case during the outbreak in 2015. As Hainan enters the post-malaria elimination stage, the significance of surveillance and response strategies cannot be overstated in preventing any resurgence of malaria and swiftly addressing potential outbreaks. Therefore, it is crucial to further strengthen surveillance systems, implement targeted response mechanisms, ensure sustainable allocation of resources, foster cross-border collaboration to curb the importation of malaria cases, monitor residual transmission hot spots, integrate these efforts with existing health systems, and prioritize research to explore innovative tools that can bolster surveillance capabilities. These activities stand as top priorities to support the initiative of Healthy Hainan Construction.

Question and Answer

24. How can these measures be tailored to the local settings based on this case study demonstrating that malaria elimination was accomplished through an innovative TLS as a tool for surveillance and response strategy for the first time?

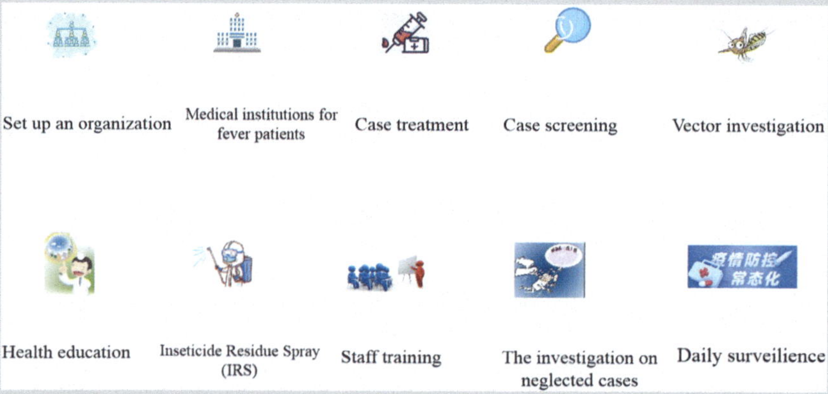

Reference answer 24:

Drawing from this case study, the following measures are recommended to tailor to local contexts using an innovative TLS for surveillance and response strategies that ultimately lead to malaria elimination:

1. Establish a dedicated committee in Sanya City to spearhead the response to the malaria epidemic. This committee will be responsible for coordinating surveillance and response efforts, and resource management in the city to ensure the effective implementation of monitoring and management tasks.
2. Strengthen the functions of fever clinics by conducting thorough investigations and blood smear examinations for patients presenting with fever symptoms.
3. Ensure that all confirmed cases are managed by the Tianya District of Sanya City and promptly transferred to the Sanya Hospital of Agricultural Reclamation, a specialized facility for treating infectious diseases, to receive standardized care.
4. Implement active case detection by screening residents in the focal villages where cases have been detected, including individuals who frequent visit forested areas.
5. Conduct thorough investigations of malaria vectors and carry out indoor residual spraying (IRS) with insecticides in the vicinity of villages where infected patients reside.
6. Launch health education campaigns by organizing household initiatives on malaria control knowledge through the Tianya District Yucai Ecological Management Committee. Engage villagers in efforts to eliminate mosquito breeding sites.
7. Provide training for medical personnel in the region to enhance their awareness and preparedness when attending to patients with fever symptoms.

8. Conduct retrospective investigations on individuals with fever to identify any instances of underreporting or concealment of cases. It is mandatory for all medical facilities in the Gaofeng area of Tianya District to conduct retrospective investigations on fever patients.
9. Establish sentinel sites such as the South Island Farm Hospital and village clinics to monitor the number of fever patients. Data from these sentinel sites, including Lixin and Baolong clinics, should be reported to Sanya CDC on a weekly basis via short message service (SMS).

Recommended discussion time:

- 3 min

25. What additional strategies, methods, or approaches could be synchronized to prevent the reestablishment of malaria transmission in the future?

Reference answer 25:

To control the reestablishment of malaria transmission in the future, the following strategies and methods can be coordinated:

- Implement the 1-3-7 approach, which emphasizes reporting cases within 1 day, conducting case investigations within 3 days, and initiating focused investigations and actions within 7 days (Cao et al. 2014).

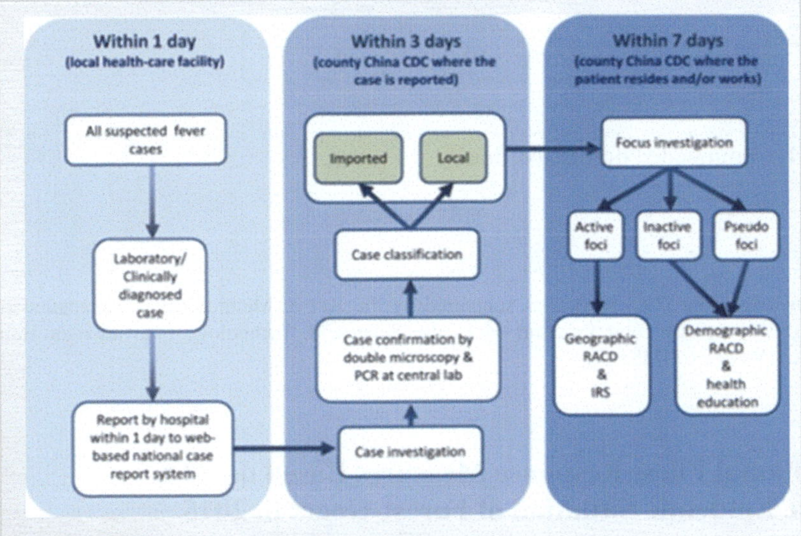

- Adopt the One Health approach, a globally recognized strategy for effectively managing emerging infectious diseases by cooperation of multisectors (Liu et al. 2022). This approach highlights the interconnected health of humans, animals, and the environment, enhancing the prevention and control of emerging zoonotic infectious diseases by bolstering health monitoring of animals, the environment, and populations at risk. This approach is renowned for its cost-effectiveness.

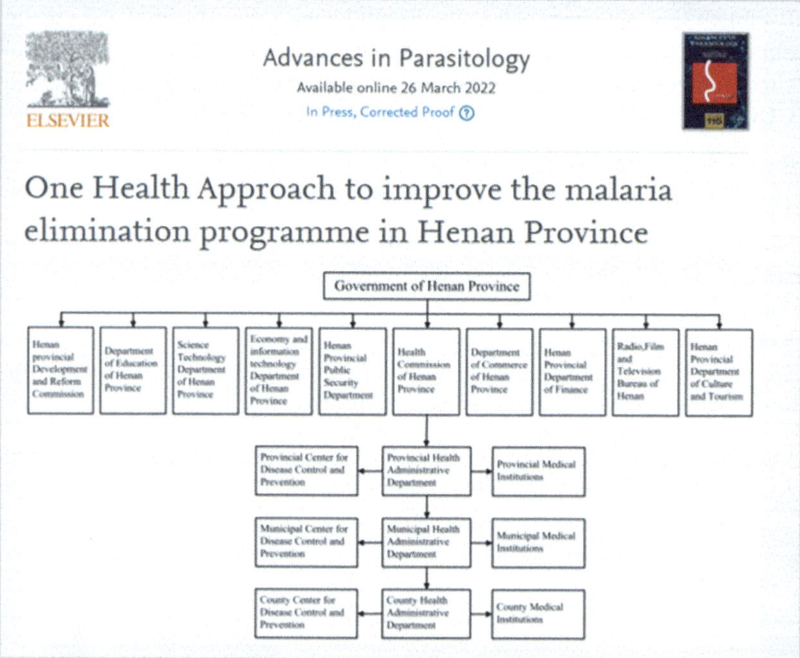

Recommended discussion time:

- 5 min

Acknowledgments This work was supported by the Bill & Melinda Gates Foundation (No. INV-018913) and by Joint Program on Health Science & Technology Innovation of Hainan Province (WSJK2024MS167).

Additional Files: Response Measures Based on TLS in the Epidemic Situation of Forest-Goers in 2015

Part 1. Methodology of the Three-Layer Strategy Implemented in Various Risk Areas

- The first layer involved the selection of three villages—Baolong, Lixin, and Zhanan in Gaofeng Township, Sanya City, and seven villages in Xinzheng Township, Baoting County (Shirang, Maowen, Xinzheng, Maopeng, Baodao,

Shenna, and Nangai) for targeted screening of the high-risk population. A total of 1823 blood slides and PCR screenings were conducted in these villages in Baoting County and Sanya City. Three positive samples were detected in blood slides, and 13 positive samples were identified through PCR. Through verification, four cases (Cases 2, 3, 4, and 6) were confirmed, while false positives were excluded. Case 5 was validated, and an outpatient was diagnosed with *P. malariae*.

The three-layer strategy conducted in the 2015 epidemic response

Layers	Names of counties or cities	Names of township	Names of village	Epidemic response in 2015				
				PCD		ACD		
				Ne.	Pos.	Ne.	Pos.	HRP[a]
1st layer	Sanya	Gaofeng	Baolong[b]	67	0	400	0	352
			Lixin[b]	74	0	558	4	530
			Zhanan[b]	35	1	684	0	394
			Shirang	58	0	17	0	15
			Maowen	45	0	5	0	5
			Xinzheng	39	0	8	0	8
	Baoting	Xinzheng	Maopeng	53	0	7	0	7
			Baodao	43	0	11	0	11
			Shenna	41	0	27	0	27
			Nangai	41	0	53	0	53

ACD active case detection, *PCD* passive case detection, *HRP* The high-risk population is defined as forest visitors among local residents and residents surrounding the focal points

[a]The number of HRPs is dynamic and too extensive to obtain in the second and third layers. However, it can be inferred from malaria parasite detection and forest visitor data

[b]Baolong village comprises four parts or natural villages including: Hongqi, Zhatao, Zhaban, Xianjin; Zhanan village is composed of seven parts or natural villages including: Nanjin, Hongxing, Jiayue, Xincun, Baotu, Ganyou, Lingqu; Lixin village includes six parts or natural villages including: Zhayun, Zhaka, Zhaye, Zhachu, Zhaye, Xincun

- The second layer encompassed the selection of ten townships including: Gaofeng Township and Yucai Township in Sanya City, Daan Township and Zhizhong Township in Ledong County, Xiangshui Township, Maogan Township, Nanlin Township, Sandao Township, Xinzhen Township in Baoting County, and Changhao Township in Wuzhishan City. Passive case detection (PCD) and active case detection (ACD) were conducted for forest visitors, primarily in Gaofeng Township and its neighboring areas. A total of 7831 blood slides were screened in the target townships, with testing carried out on all individuals visiting the forests.

The three-layer strategy conducted in the 2015 epidemic response								
Layers	Names of counties or cities	Names of township	Names of village	Epidemic response in 2015				
				PCD		ACD		
				Ne.	Pos.	Ne.	Pos.	HRP[a]
2nd layer	Sanya	Gaofeng[b]		1216	0	0	0	–
		Yucai		1109	0	553	0	–
		Daan		83	0	317	0	–
	Ledong	Zhizhong		548	0	32	0	–
		Baoguo		82	0	447	0	–
	Baoting	Xiangshui		331	0	103	0	–
		Maogan		350	0	0	0	–
		Nanlin		600	0	258	0	–
		Xinzheng[b]		742	0	0	0	–
		Sandao		740	0	0	0	–
	Wuzhishan	Changhao		320	0	0	0	–

ACD active case detection, *PCD* passive case detection, *HRP* The high-risk population is defined as forest visitors among local residents and residents surrounding the focal points

[a]The number of HRPs is dynamic and too extensive to obtain in the second and third layers. However, it can be inferred from malaria parasite detection and forest visitor data

[b]The data from the previous layer are indicated. A single dash denotes unavailable information

– In the third layer, 12 counties or cities—Ledong, Baoting, Wuzhishan, Dongfang, Lingshui, Qiongzhong, Baisha, Changjiang, Wanning, Qionghai, Tunchang, and Danzhou—were chosen. Health education initiatives for communities and passive case detection for forest visitors were primarily conducted around Sanya City and its surrounding areas. A total of 95,350 blood slides were screened in the targeted townships, with testing administered to all individuals visiting the forests.

The three-layer strategy conducted in the 2015 epidemic response

Layers	Names of counties or cities	Names of township	Names of village	Epidemic response in 2015				
				PCD		ACD		
				Ne.	Pos.	Ne.	Pos.	HRP[a]
3rd layer	Sanya[b]			11,039	0	15	0	–
	Ledong			4261	0	4332	0	–
	Baoting[b]			5529	0	142	0	–
	Wuzhishan			2120	0	885	0	–
	Dongfang			9496	0	0	0	–
	Lingshui			5359	0	1747	0	–
	Qiongzhong			3427	0	2640	0	–
	Baisha			6828	0	588	0	–
	Changjiang			2294	0	2293	0	–
	Waning			9354	0	1115	0	–
	Qionghai			5582	0	1624	0	–
	Tunchang			1969	0	1626	0	–
	Danzhou			10,297	0	158	0	–
Total				84,172	1	21,328	4	1422

ACD active case detection, *PCD* passive case detection, *HRP* The high-risk population is defined as forest visitors among local residents and residents surrounding the focal points

[a]The number of HRPs is dynamic and too extensive to obtain in the second and third layers. However, it can be inferred from malaria parasite detection and forest visitor data

[b]The data from the previous layer are indicated. A single dash denotes unavailable information

Part 2. Vector Surveillance and Control Measures in Three-Layer Risk Areas

- In the first layer, vector surveillance and control measures were implemented to facilitate the elimination of focal points and mitigate transmission risks. According to the 2015 dynamic vector surveillance outcomes in the three layers, *An. minimus* and *An. sinensis* mosquitoes were captured in the first layer in Sanya City, with *An. sinensis* emerging as the predominant species (Fig. 3.5).
- In the second layer, *An. minimus* and *An. dirus* were exclusively identified in Wuzhishan City, while *An. sinensis* continued to dominate (Fig. 3.5).

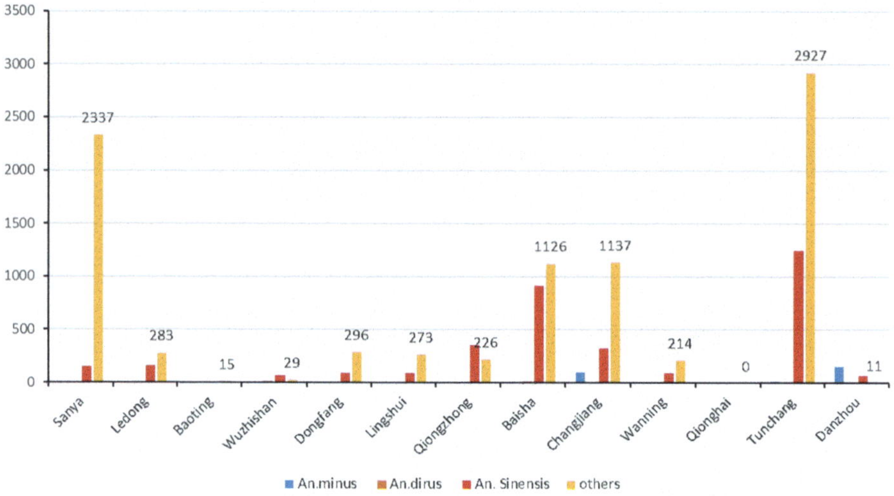

Fig. 3.5 The number of mosquitoes detected through vector surveillance in the risk areas segmented by the three-layer approach

- In the third layer, *An. minimus* was detected in Changjiang County, Danzhou City, Baisha County, and Tunchang County, while *An. dirus* was present in Baisha County. *An. sinensis*, on the other hand, was prevalent in all counties except for Qionghai City. These findings highlight the existence of highly efficient malaria vectors in Sanya City, where the focal villages are located. Furthermore, significant malaria vectors persisted in specific counties or cities within Hainan Province, underscoring the necessity for continuous surveillance efforts to monitor vector dynamics (Fig. 3.5).

Part 3. Distribution of Mosquito Nets in Three-Layered Risk Areas

Indoor residual spraying (IRS) with deltamethrin was solely executed in the first layer, while LLINs were distributed and utilized across the three layers, encompassing most counties or cities except for Tunchang County and Wanning City (Fig. 3.6).

Note: *The data regarding IRS were not provided, and IRS activities were exclusively carried out in Sanya to address six focal points.

Part 4. Training Activities in Three-Layered Risk Areas

Training sessions were conducted for clinicians, public health personnel, and researchers to enhance preparedness for the outbreak in 2015 (Fig. 3.7).

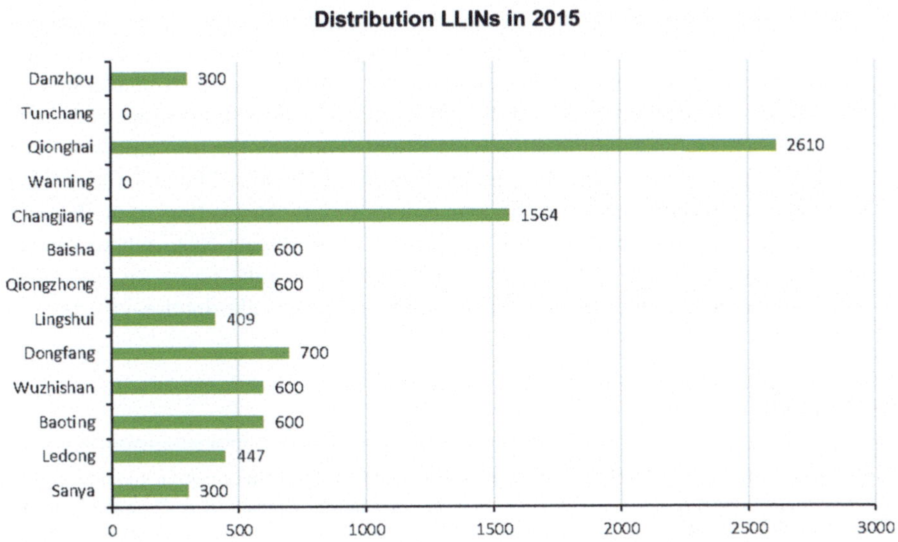

Fig. 3.6 The number of long-lasting insecticidal nets (LLINs) delivered in the risk areas categorized by the three-layer approach

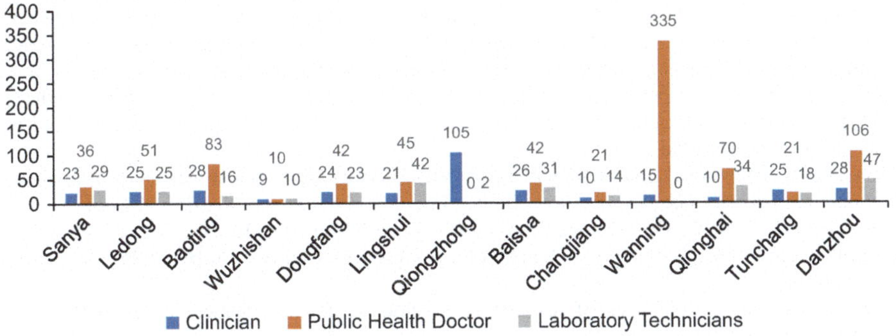

Fig. 3.7 The number of individuals who underwent training in the risk areas segmented by the three-layer approach

Part 5. Results and Conclusions

– Patients were treated with chloroquine phosphate tablets/primaquine phosphate tablets (each tablet containing chloroquine phosphate 0.25 g and primaquine phosphate 13.2 mg). After an 8-day treatment course, they were discharged from the hospital, and subsequent regular follow-up rapid diagnostic tests (RDT) showed negative results. No relapses occurred, and the patients have since resumed their normal work and daily routines.

- The three-level system (TLS) is effective for outbreaks originating from indigenous cases of unknown origin or isolated cases lacking comprehensive epidemic data. Conversely, the 1-3-7 approach is well-suited for isolated cases with clear epidemic indicators, such as imported cases and individuals in close proximity to imported cases.
- The TLS represents a significant advancement following the implementation of the 1-3-7 approach in eradicating malaria during outbreaks. The innovative TLS methodology has proven to be effective among the forest-dwellers in the Hainan case study and holds promise for application in Southeast Asia, where forest-dwellers constitute a high-risk group, and malaria transmission by *An. dirus* and *An. minimus* mosquitoes presents a challenge to malaria elimination efforts.

References

Cao J, Sturrock HJ, Cotter C, Zhou S, Zhou H, Liu Y et al (2014) Communicating and monitoring surveillance and response activities for malaria elimination: China's "1-3-7" strategy. PLoS Med 11(5):e1001642

Li YC, Wang SQ, Hu XM, Huang YJ, Chen RQ, Lin MC, Xu HZ, Ye RS, Zhan DT, Huang SL, Zhen J, Wen XD, Wang GY, Liu Y, Li HS, Zheng ZC, Wang J, Zeng W, Meng F, Huang XM, Wang GZ, Yang B, Chen Y (2022a) Surveillance and response systems driving malaria elimination in the mountain areas of Hainan province. Adv Parasitol 116:69

Li Y, Huang Y, Chen R, Huang W, Xu H, Ye R, Huang S, Zhen J, Wen X, Wang G, Liu Y, Li H, Zheng Z, Wang J, Wang G, Chen C, Zeng W, Meng F, Huang X, Wang G, Yang B, Chen Y (2022b) An innovative three-layer strategy in response to a quartan malaria outbreak among forest goers in Hainan Island, China: a retrospective study. Infect Dis Poverty11(1):97

Lin M, Chen S, Deng J, Si Y, Zhong H, Huang M, Chen X, Cao R (1993) Investigation on malaria infection among residents of forest goers accommodation in high malaria area of Hainan Province. Hainan Med J 4:8–9

Lin C, Chen Z, Wang S, Luo P, Wu D, Zheng A, Wei J (2016) Analysis and management of a rare malaria case of *P. malariae* in Sanya, Hainan Province. Chin J Trop Med 165:481–484

Liu Y, He ZQ, Wang D, Hu YB, Qian D, Yang CY, Zhou RM, Li SH, Lu DL, Zhang HW (2022) One health approach to improve the malaria elimination programme in Henan Province. Adv Parasitol 116:153

Wei S, Lin S, Yang C (2007) The 50-year history of health service development in Hainan Province from 1950 to 2000. Nanfang Press, Haikou

Xia ZG, Zhang L, Feng J, Li M, Feng XY, Tang LH, Wang SQ, Yang HL, Gao Q, Kramer R, Ernest T, Yap P, Zhou XN (2014) Lessons from malaria control to elimination: case study in Hainan and Yunnan provinces. Adv Parasitol 86:47–79

Yin JH, Zhou SS, Xia ZG, Wang RB, Qian YJ, Yang WZ, Zhou XN (2014) Historical patterns of malaria transmission in China. Adv Parasitol 86:1–19

Zhou SS, Zhang SS, Zhang L, Rietveld AE, Ramsay AR, Zachariah R, Bissell K, Van Den Bergh R, Xia ZG, Zhou XN, Cibulskis RE (2015) China's 1-3-7 surveillance and response strategy for malaria elimination: is case reporting, investigation and foci response happening according to plan? Infect Dis Poverty 4:55

Chapter 4
How to Ensure the Effect of Mass Drug Administration (MDA) on the Control of *Plasmodium vivax* Malaria

Xian Xu, Jian-Jun Wang, Wei-Dong Li, Tao Zhang, Jing-Jing Jiang, Xiao-Feng Lv, and Shu-Qi Wang

Learning Objectives
Through this case, students will be able to:

1. Understand the effectiveness of mass drug administration (MDA) on the control of vivax malaria.
2. Understand the necessary conditions for the implementation of MDA.
3. Understand essential factors contributing to the success of MDA.
4. Understand how to ensure the effectiveness of MDA.

This case is provided by the Anhui Provincial Center for Disease Control and Prevention, implemented in Anhui Province from 2007 to 2014 and compiled in 2022 and 2023.

4.1 Part 1. Background

Anhui Province is in the eastern part of China, with an area of 140,100 km^2. There are 16 prefecture-level cities, with a total resident population of 61.13 million at the end of 2022 (Xu and Zhang 2022). Historically, Anhui Province has been a serious malaria-endemic province in China, where *vivax* malaria is the dominant species (Xu et al. 2020). The terrain of Anhui Province is divided into mountainous areas, hills, and plains from south to north. Typically, malaria is transmitted between May and October. The last malaria outbreak in Anhui Province occurred in 2006, and 34,984 cases were reported, with an incidence rate of 5.72/10,000 (Zhou et al.

X. Xu · J.-J. Wang · W.-D. Li (✉) · T. Zhang · J.-J. Jiang · X.-F. Lv · S.-Q. Wang
Anhui Provincial Center for Disease Control and Prevention,
Hefei, Anhui, People's Republic of China

X.-N. Zhou, J.-H. Yin (eds.), *Malaria Control and Elimination in China*,
https://doi.org/10.1007/978-981-97-8719-7_4

2007). These cases were mainly distributed in the rural parts of 24 counties in 6 prefecture-level cities on the Huaibei Plain.

Question and Answer

1. What measures should be taken to control an outbreak of malaria?

Answer:

1. Individual treatment.
2. Mass drug administration.
3. Mosquito control (indoor residual spraying).
4. Personal protection.

According to the Emergency Treatment Plan for Malaria issued by the Ministry of Health of the People's Republic of China in 2006, on-site management of *vivax* malaria outbreaks includes the following:

1. Individual treatment: Standardized antimalarial treatment should be provided promptly for all suspected, clinically diagnosed, and confirmed cases of malaria, with an 8-day strategy of chloroquine (substrate) at a total dose of 1.2 g for 3 days for adults and additional primaquine (substrate) at a total dose of 180 mg for 8 days for adults.
2. Mass drug administration (MDA) for prevention: Piperaquine (600 mg) or chloroquine (0.3 g) should be given to the family members and neighbors of patients according to their condition in towns and villages with an incidence rate of malaria greater than 10%. If necessary, preventive administration can be conducted for all people in a town, village, or village group.
3. Vector control: When the density of *Anopheles* mosquitoes increases abnormally, relevant measures should be taken. To kill mosquitoes, pyrethroid insecticides can be used to spray houses where people and livestock staying and to deliver the insecticide-treated nets (ITN) around the whole town, village, or village group. The recommended dose of pyrethroid insecticides used to soak or spray a mosquito net is 20–30 mg/m^2.
4. Personal protection: Measures that reduce contact between people and mosquitoes, such as correct mosquito net use and sleeping indoors, should be taught to the public (Xia et al. 2014).

In 2007, the People's Government of Anhui Province decided to implement a wide range of MDA (MDA in a specific range), which delineated the range of MDA based on malaria cases and the distribution of water bodies in a natural village. From 2008 to 2015, MDA in a specific range was conducted in all natural villages in the province that experienced malaria cases in the past 2 years (Xu et al. 2022).

4.2 Part 2 Implementation of MDA

Question and Answer
2. What are the requirements for MDA?
Answer:

1. Formulation of a technical plan for MDA and determination of the range and object of administration, the type and dosage of the drugs, and the administration timeline.
2. A guaranteed supply of the medicine.
3. Government support and policy approval.
4. High rates of acceptance among participants.

MDA is a powerful and effective measure used to control the malaria epidemic based on China's historical prevention and control experiences. Before implementing MDA, it is necessary to determine which antimalarial drugs to use first, clarify the drug supply method by performing market research to identify pharmaceutical factories or companies that can provide the necessary amount of drugs, and obtain government support and funding for the purchase of drugs. In China, antimalaria medicine for MDA is distributed free of charge. For example, in 2007, the People's Government of Anhui Province allocated 4.8 million yuan to purchase piperaquine phosphate tablets for 4.2 million people. At the same time, MDA should be implemented in regions and populations that permit MDA in accordance with local policies, customs, and religions. Ultimately, acceptance of the project by MDA participants should be promoted through various measures.

Question and Answer
3. How can drug regimens for MDA for the control of *vivax* malaria be determined?
Answer:

Appropriate drugs should be chosen based on their antimalarial mechanisms and half-life. In addition, it is crucial to determine the optimal timing for drug administration in relation to the malaria transmission period.

Experts selected different types, dosages, dosing intervals, and treatment durations of MDA drugs based on regional and temporal factors. In Anhui Province, from 2008 to 2014, a regimen of 180 mg primaquine phosphate (PQ) was implemented before the transmission season. Adults took a daily dose of 22.5 mg for 8 consecutive days, usually from January to March. PQ is the only widely used drug that targets the dormant intrahepatic stage of *P. vivax*. However, it can cause severe side effects, such as hemolytic anemia, in individuals with G6PD deficiency. Therefore, MDA is prohibited for people with this condition.

Question and Answer

4. How does the government support the implementation of MDA?

Answer:

Organizational guarantees, funding guarantees, and institutional guarantees

Strong organizational support is the key to the success of MDA. Before each implementation of MDA, Anhui Province established work organizations at the provincial, municipal, county, and rural levels and signed target responsibility agreements at all levels. Leadership groups, technical guidance groups, and supervision groups were established at the provincial and municipal levels; leadership groups, medication scope delineation groups, and supervision groups were established at the county level; and leadership groups and medication delivery teams were established at the rural level (Fig. 4.1).

To ensure the effective implementation of MDA, national, provincial, municipal, county, and township governments allocated special funds, along with funds from the malaria project granted by the Global Fund Against HIV/AIDS, Tubculosis and Malaria, to finance the following activities: purchasing drugs, organizing training courses, promoting and mobilizing, providing work subsidies for medication delivery teams, and supervising transportation for the leadership team (Fig. 4.2).

In terms of institutional guarantees, a supervision and assessment system was established, and on-site supervision, patrol supervision, and telephone inquiries

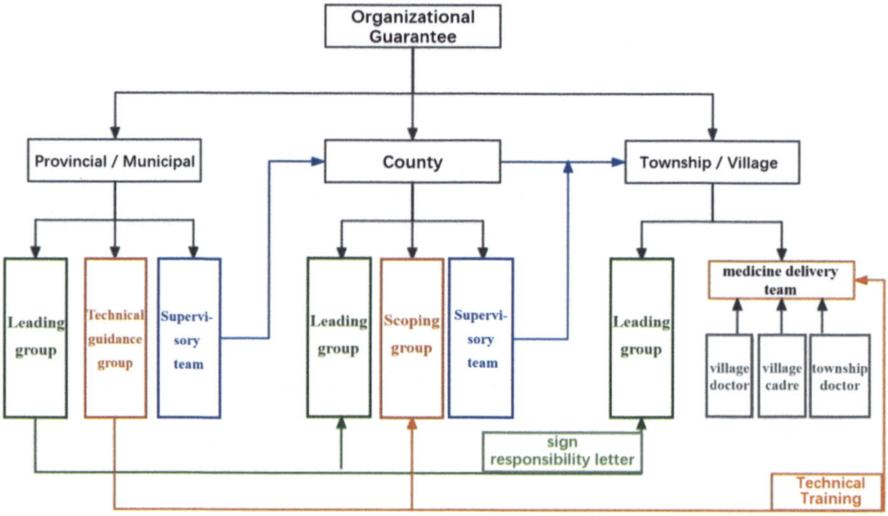

Fig. 4.1 Organizational guarantees of MDA in Anhui Province

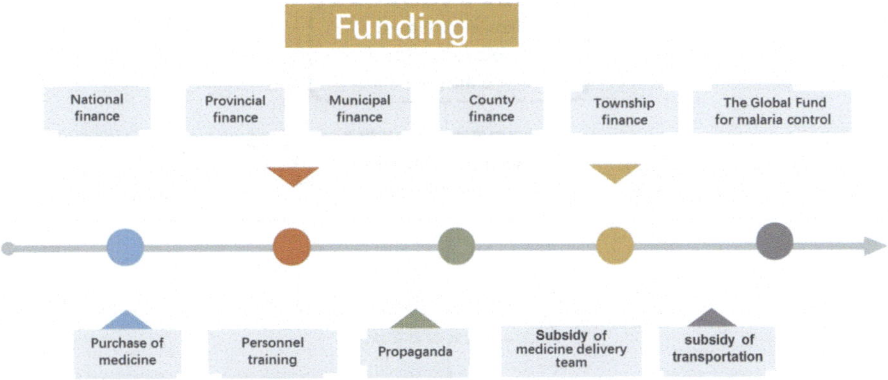

Fig. 4.2 The diagram for funding guarantee of MDA in Anhui Province

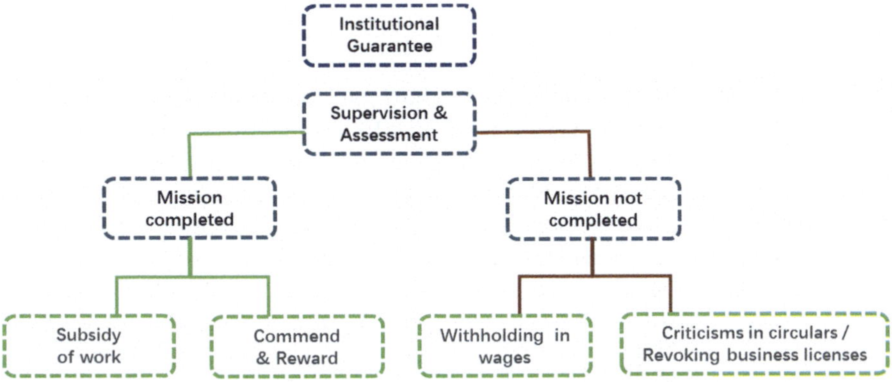

Fig. 4.3 The diagram for institutional guarantees of MDA in Anhui Province

were organized by stationed and touring supervision teams at the provincial, municipal, and county levels. Work subsidies are provided to medication delivery teams to reward organizations and individuals who excel in their work. For those who do not complete their work, in addition to requesting additional tasks, salaries may be deducted, and the business license of the village clinic may even be revoked (Fig. 4.3).

Question and Answer

5. What are the essential factors contributing to the success of MDA?

Answer:

Technical training, registration, drug distribution, and publicity and mobilization.

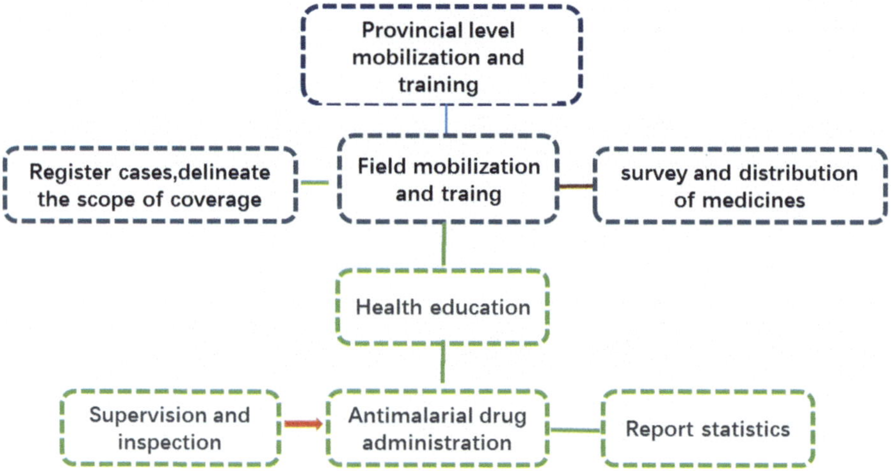

Fig. 4.4 The specific steps involved in implementing MDA in Anhui Province

Figure 4.4 shows the specific steps of MDA implementation. After the medication plan is formulated, provincial-level mobilization and training meetings are held. Each natural village that receives medication conducts a thorough registration of cases, defines the scope of medication, and performs layer-by-layer mobilization and training of medication workers in cities, counties, and townships. Medication is considered officially implemented after drugs are distributed from the provincial level to the village level. Supervision and inspection are carried out throughout the entire process. Finally, any gaps are identified and filled, and statistics are reported.

In Anhui, in the MDA protocol document, the provincial health administrative department requires that before any region implements MDA, it must firstly register a list of people within the range of MDA, document the type and number of people who need medicine, survey the existing conditions for carrying out health education within the administration range, and organize and train the staff involved in health education. Staff members participating in the project from various regions include health workers from counties, towns, and villages; village cadres; and teachers. All towns and villages are required to carry out various forms of health education activities according to local conditions and arrange special funds for health education. Before each MDA, the provincial government should formulate a working plan for the year and organize provincial technical training courses for cities and counties. The municipal and county governments should organize mobilization meetings and technical training courses for health workers in towns and villages, and drugs should be distributed from the province, cities, counties, and towns to all administrative villages.

Provincial-level professional and technical personnel formulate specific administration technical plans that clarify the range and objective of administration, the type and dosage of the drugs, the administration time frame, and the goal administration rate, which is determined through preliminary investigations and experiments. The provincial health administrative department issues a document to clarify the organizational guarantees in various regions, including the funding guarantee, personnel guarantee, and system guarantee. The provincial health administrative department also arranges the timing and formulates the requirements for administration technical training, drug distribution, and publicity and mobilization at all levels and regions. All counties are required to carry out MDA simultaneously within the specified time frame.

Question and Answer

6. What challenges may be faced during MDA, and what are the corresponding measures?

Answer:

1. Organizational integrity of the administration (assigning an individual/a team to be responsible for one district; administration supervision).
2. Compliance of administration subjects (health education).
3. Measures for adverse drug reactions (administration plan, precautions, and adverse reaction treatment plan).
4. Availability of administration subjects (targeted delivery method and time).

In the MDA process, there are two main types of personnel involved. One is staff, including medication delivery teams, adverse drug reaction handling staff, and technical instructors. Staff should be skilled and sufficient in number. As part of the MDA process in Anhui Province, a medication delivery team is responsible for the daily door-to-door delivery of medication to each recipient. Usually, each administrative village has one or several medication delivery teams. Other parts of the MDA process include the immediate treatment of adverse drug reactions by the adverse drug reaction handling staff, delineation of the administration range of each natural village, determination of the administration subjects, and control of the administration quality by the technical instructors throughout the whole process.

The other type of personnel is the administration staff. The administration staff should be highly compliant with the MDA work. How can high levels of compliance be achieved? Effective health education is needed to help staff understand the benefits of the medicine, why the medicine is necessary, who needs to take the medicine, how to obtain the medicine, when to take the medicine, and what precautions should be taken. Informing people in this manner improves the likelihood that they will follow the instructions of the medicine delivery team. Moreover, the delivery method and time must be arranged according to the availability of the administration subjects. This can be achieved through communication after the patients receive effective health education and demonstrate willingness to comply with the recommendations.

Question and Answer
7. How can MDA drugs be delivered in Anhui Province?
Answer:

Directly observed therapy (DOT)

The medication delivery team in each village went door-to-door every day to the homes of residents, delivered the drugs, and supervised the residents as they took the drugs. This direct supervised treatment method is known as the directly observed therapy (DOT) method. The DOT method can encourage compliance with medication and improve the safety of MDA by enabling direct observation of possible adverse drug reactions.

Question and Answer
8. Who should serve as the drug delivery staff?
Answer:

Professional people with characteristics such as public appeal, authority, and accessibility.

When selecting professionals, it is necessary to consider both the quantity needed and the requirements of the specific implementation work. When selecting personnel for specific work, the following principles should be followed:

1. *Professionalism*. Due to the importance of professional knowledge, skills, and practical experience, personnel should be selected from professional institutions, such as local health institutions. Before they start work, they need to be uniformly trained. Centralized training for village doctors and village officials plays a crucial role in ensuring the quality of MDA. It is essential that all personnel involved in the program understand the requirements and adhere to them strictly. Prior to the commencement of MDA implementation in 2007, the Anhui Provincial Centers for Disease Control and Prevention (CDC) organized a training course for the implementation plan in Anhui Province. Subsequently, seven groups organized by the provincial CDC conducted field training in 22 key counties, focusing on the implementation plan and the method of delineating the medication coverage area. Technical guidance teams were established at the provincial, prefectural, and county levels to provide training to staff before implementation. Provincial-level officials conducted face-to-face technical training at the county level, covering various aspects such as delineating the coverage area, identifying eligible recipients, recognizing contraindications, managing adverse drug reactions, and completing medication records. At the county level, professionals were trained to delineate the coverage area in each natural village and to educate medication delivery teams on medication techniques. This ensured that

personnel at all levels understood the program requirements and adhered to them strictly. In subsequent years, provincial-level training was cascaded down to the prefectural level, followed by training for township and village staff at the county level.

2. *Public appeal*. Public appeal refers to professional personnel who are popular among the public. This enables them to successfully deliver drugs and popularize health science.
3. *Authority*. An authoritative person may be more convincing.
4. Accessibility and convenient short-distance commutes.

Village cadres and doctors in rural areas, who are locally influential and appealing, are suitable staff for MDA; principals and head teachers can be selected in schools. In addition, local experienced and prestigious volunteers can be selected. It is necessary to exclude those who are not sufficiently responsible.

The medication delivery teams in each village in Anhui include three to five staff members, comprising mainly township doctors, village cadres, and village doctors.

Question and Answer
9. What is the optimal timing for drug administration?
Answer:

Certain times of day are more suitable for drug delivery and monitoring adverse drug reactions.

To minimize the occurrence of adverse reactions and prevent gastrointestinal discomfort resulting from taking medication on an empty stomach, some towns implemented centralized drug delivery periods following breakfast and lunch.

Question and Answer
10. Why is health education necessary to conduct MDA?
Answer:

1. MDA relies on the voluntary participation of the population.
2. Participants need to know why and how to take the medicine and understand the precautions.
3. The purpose of health education is to enable participants to take the medicine as needed voluntarily and achieve the ultimate goal of controlling the source of infection.

Accepting medicine is voluntary, and informed consent needs to be obtained from the administration subjects before the MDA process is carried out. To facilitate participation, educators must help people understand the importance of taking the medicine, the proper method for taking the medicine, and any precautions. The goal is for everyone participating in MDA to take the medicine, so that the source of infection is eliminated and the epidemic is controlled.

Question and Answer

11. What are the characteristics of health education for MDA compared with general health education?

Answer:

1. MDA education is short, is conducted before and during administration, and concludes when administration is finished.
2. Implementation is urgently needed.
3. The effects can appear immediately after the participant takes the medicine.

The specific periods for MDA designed to control the *vivax* malaria epidemic in Anhui Province included August, September, and October 2007; April 2008; and January 2009–2015. In 2007, three tablets of piperaquine phosphate were taken orally for an adult once a month for 3 months during the malaria epidemic, whereas in 2008 and after, three tablets of primaquine phosphate were taken orally daily for 8 consecutive days during the dormant stage of malaria. Therefore, the corresponding health education program lasted for a short time and was implemented only during the preparation and administration periods. For example, education was carried out from July to October 2007, including the month of administration and the month prior, and concluded after administration. Because malaria is not a chronic disease, the purpose of MDA is to control the epidemic quickly. Therefore, health education is most urgent. To ensure the quality of administration, we require all counties involved to start administrative work on a fixed date, and health education must commence immediately after the administration plan is issued. The effect of health education is reflected by the administration rate; a high rate can indicate effective health education, while a low rate shows that health education and other work to enhance the rate need to be improved.

Question and Answer

12. What is the core malaria-related information that needs to be promoted via the health education aspect of MDA?

Answer:

The reoccurrence and severity of malaria, the importance of taking medicine, how to take the medicine, precautions, and possible adverse reactions.

The basic requirements for health information include the following:

1. Pertinence and science of the content.
2. Accurate and universal use of symbols suitable for the audience and media.

3. Proper expression to meet publicity goals.

Core information refers to the information disseminated to the target population. The steps used to determine the core information include the following:

1. Listing the information needs according to the target population and health-related issues.
2. Determining the expected changes in behavior.
3. Determining practical behaviors.
4. Analyzing factors related to practical behavioral patterns.
5. Selecting information that can help the target population change its behavior.

The core information that needs to be promoted to all administration subjects includes the following:

1. The definition of malaria and the epidemic situation in the area in recent years. Malaria is a parasitic disease transmitted by mosquito bites.
2. The severity of malaria. Malaria causes chills, fever, anemia, and jaundice, and in some severe cases, death may occur.
3. The importance of MDA. Malaria epidemics are highly sporadic along and north of the Huai River in Anhui Province. Conditions in some areas are exacerbated rapidly, as no signs or symptoms are present in a considerable number of people who may have been infected with malaria parasites. This becomes an "invisible" source of infection. MDA for patients with malaria can eliminate the source of infection and prevent the onset and spread of malaria.
4. How to take the medicine. Because of the regionality and regularity of the incidence of malaria, local health and anti-epidemic personnel will delimit a certain area where all residents will take the medicine. For example, during the MDA project in the dormant stage in 2008, three tablets of primaquine were administered once a day for 8 days, resulting in a total of 24 tablets for adults; for children, the dosage was decreased according to age. The general public is requested to cooperate with antimalarial treatment in the dormant stage under the guidance of local health personnel. Only when individuals cooperate can they, their family, and their neighbors avoid contracting malaria and stop its spread.
5. Precautions. (1) The medicine must be taken according to the prescribed dose and preferably after meals. (2) Those who are under 1 year old, pregnant women, breastfeeding women, elderly individuals, frail individuals, and those with chronic cardiovascular diseases or liver or kidney dysfunction should not take the drug.
6. Possible side effects. The side effects of this drug are minor. A few patients may have anorexia, upper abdominal discomfort, vomiting, abdominal pain, cramps, or dizziness. Abdominal cramps or neutropenia may occur occasionally. When a serious reaction occurs, the local medical institution should be contacted.

Question and Answer
13. What are the characteristics of each group of health education subjects? Which group should be chosen as the key group?
Answer:

It is necessary to analyze the groups into which the subjects of health education can be divided, as well as the general condition and behavioral characteristics of each group, such as their activity scope, education level, and time available for health education.

The target population of health education refers to the target or specific group that receives the health education intervention, that is, the population that expects to change its behavior, the direct beneficiaries of health education, and the target population of the current MDA. The population affected by malaria caused by MDA in Anhui Province is located in the northern rural area of the province and can be divided into young adults, women, children, and elderly people according to age and sex. According to the survey, 30%–40% of the local population works in more economically developed provinces, such as Zhejiang, Jiangsu, and Shanghai. They are mainly male young adults and adults ages 18–55 years who go home for the Spring Festival (January to February) and engage in farming during the wheat harvest (June–July). Women, children, and elderly people mostly stay at home year-round. Most of the women who stay at home are engaged in housework and farming and are at home at noon and in the evening, and most elderly people stay at home or walk around in the village throughout the day. Preschool-age children have a similar activity scope to that of elderly individuals; most school-age children go to school in the village or town, so they stay at home at noon and night, and a few of them go to school in the county or city, so they stay at home on weekends. A small number of young men and women who work near their homes go out early and return late every day.

The two key groups of this health education program were defined as women and students, according to activity scope and educational level, combined with time available for health education. Because the health of women affects the health of their family members, especially their children, health education for women is an important facet of the population's health education. Students were regarded as a key group because of the ongoing development and plasticity of their mind and body, their curiosity, their thirst for knowledge, and their role as mentors to younger students.

Question and Answer

14. What are the appropriate health education methods for different target groups?

Answer:

Because their education typically includes elementary or junior high school, most women have a vocabulary that comprises commonly used words. Therefore, health education can be promoted through various approaches, especially the distribution of daily necessities.

For students, because of their understanding of commonly used words and high level of acceptance of health education, health education can be promoted through various approaches. Students are also willing to accept school supplies.

Most elderly individuals have a relatively low education level; therefore, verbal communication is recommended. This includes verbally presented introductions from staff, family members, and others.

Young adults mostly read at a junior high school level; therefore, they can understand mandarin and recognize Chinese characters, so various approaches can be used for health education.

Different target groups have different levels of acceptance of different health education methods. For example, health education for women should be carried out in accordance with physical, psychological, educational, and environmental characteristics; most rural women in the northern Anhui Province have an elementary or junior high school education level; therefore, they can recognize most commonly used words, and various health education methods can be applied. In addition, since women are mainly engaged in housework, they are most willing to accept the distribution of daily necessities. Because students understand commonly used words and have a high level of acceptance of health education, multiple methods and media can be used to attract their attention. Due to physical and educational limitations, elderly people require more attention. They can obtain information by listening to staff and family members. Young adults were not listed as a key population in this health education program, since most of them work outside the province, where there is poor accessibility. However, they have a better physical condition, greater scope of daily activities, and higher literacy level. They understand Mandarin and recognize characters. Thus, health education can be promoted through various methods. In addition, due to their high level of acceptance of information, health education has a greater effect on this population than on others.

MDA is mainly carried out in rural areas. The conditions for health education in these areas were as follows: each administrative village had a village committee and a village clinic, and in larger administrative villages, there were rural primary schools. Most administrative villages were equipped with large loudspeakers outdoors, and villagers had televisions in their homes. Each villager's house was independent, consisting of a one-story bungalow or a two-story small building with a cement brick structure.

The health education methods adopted by the Anhui Provincial Government in an effort to improve MDA compliance included the following activities:

1. Media promotion: Broadcast news reports, special films, and slogans on official television and radio.
2. Banner promotion: Hung, pasted, or painted malaria prevention and control slogans on the exterior walls of villages and roadside residential buildings.
3. Promotional cartoons in schools.
4. Promotion by the village head through the village radio station.
5. Distributed health education products with promotional knowledge points, such as family aprons, calendar paintings, mosquito screen doors, shopping bags, visual acuity charts for students, exercise books, and pens. Local dialects, parallel sentences, and rhymes were used for these products.

Question and Answer
15. What is the level of acceptance of these health education products? Which are the most popular?
Answer:

Through visits and special interviews, it was determined that there are four products with the highest level of public acceptance, including public wall characters, publicity by prestigious people with loudspeakers, cartoons for students, and aprons for residents.

Figure 4.5 shows the four types of health education products with the highest level of public acceptance during MDA in Anhui Province, including public wall characters, aprons for residents, publicity by prestigious people with loudspeakers, and cartoons for students. Popular health education products may differ according to differences in economic conditions and education levels in different regions at different times.

Question and Answer
16. How can health education be used to reduce and prevent adverse drug reactions?
Answer:

All localities are required to carry out various publicity activities for the administration participants, distribute the *Health Education* paper containing the core information, conduct face-to-face communication, and obtain informed consent before participants take the medicine.

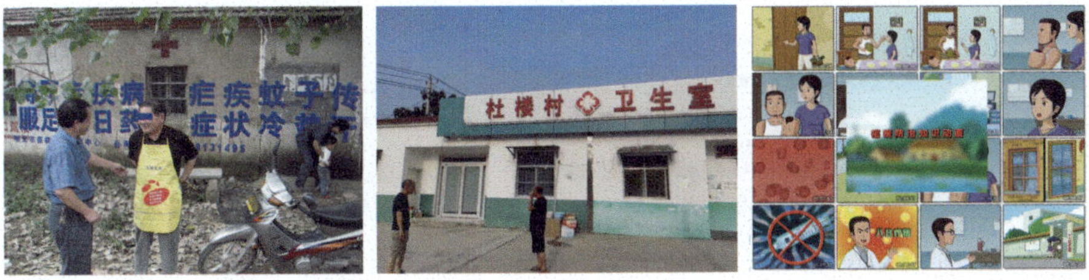

Fig. 4.5 Different types of health education products

Only after obtaining the consent of the medication recipient can medication administration be conducted. Each individual receiving medication in Anhui Province was provided with a health education prescription containing essential information about antimalarial drugs, along with cautions regarding potential side effects like anorexia, epigastric discomfort, and vomiting. The consultation phone number of the local disease prevention and control agency was provided, through which participants could receive answers to questions about any related problems in a timely manner. The prescription also featured an informed consent column that required the informed consent and signatures of the participants (Fig. 4.6a). All health education prescriptions were issued by the staff door-to-door, and some rural households placed the paper in a prominent position on the walls of their homes (Fig. 4.6b).

Medical institutions at all levels were also used as units in response to the adverse reaction. Severe reactions included cyanosis accompanied by dizziness, chest tightness, palpitations, shortness of breath, and other hypoxic symptoms, as well as severe poisoning or allergic reactions. The treatment methods for adverse reactions were provided in advance. During the transmission season in 2007, a small number of people who had received piperaquine phosphate reported mild side effects, such as dizziness, nausea, and numbness (Gou et al. 2008). A total of 719 people in the province experienced serious adverse reactions, but no poisoning cases or deaths occurred. Likewise, no deaths occurred during the MDA from 2008 to 2015.

Question and Answer

17. How can the quality of MDA be controlled?

Answer:

By providing high-quality on-site guidance and supervision.

During the implementation of MDA, county-level health professionals and health administrative personnel were responsible for guiding and supervising the work in each village. The former scientifically and reasonably delineated the scope of MDA while considering technical contraindications and precautions; the latter participated in management. On-site supervision, touring supervision, telephone

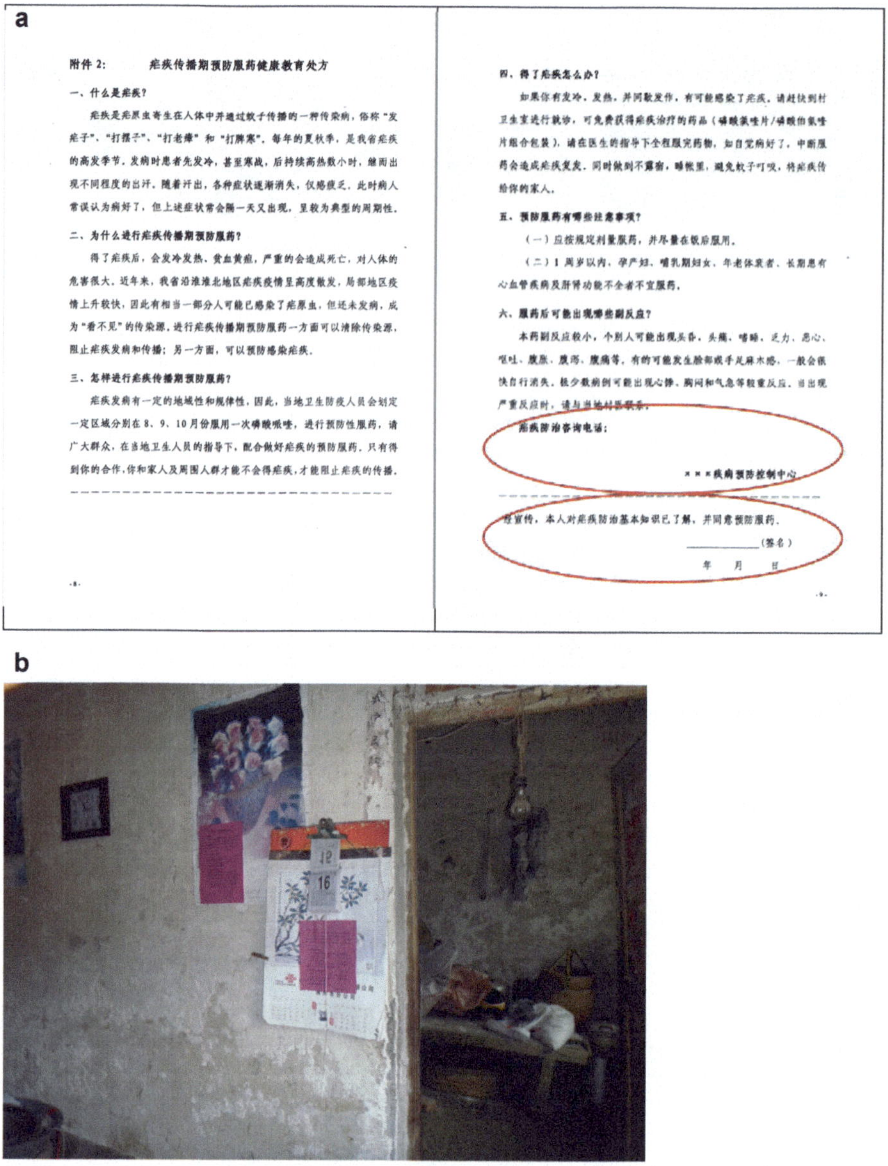

附件 2: 疟疾传播期预防服药健康教育处方

一、什么是疟疾?

疟疾是疟原虫寄生在人体中并通过蚊子传播的一种传染病，俗称"发疟子"、"打摆子"、"打老瘴"和"打脾寒"。每年的夏秋季，是我省疟疾的高发季节。发病时患者先发冷，甚至寒战，后持续高热数小时，继而出现不同程度的出汗。随着汗出，各种症状逐渐消失，仅感疲乏。此时病人常误认为病好了，但上述症状常会隔一天又出现，呈较为典型的周期性。

二、为什么进行疟疾传播期预防服药?

得了疟疾后，会发冷发热、贫血黄疸，严重的会造成死亡，对人体的危害很大。近年来，我省沿淮淮北地区疟疾疫情呈高度散发，局部地区疫情上升较快，因此有相当一部分人可能已感染了疟原虫，但还未发病，成为"看不见"的传染源。进行疟疾传播期预防服药一方面可以清除传染源，阻止疟疾发病和传播；另一方面，可以预防感染疟疾。

三、怎样进行疟疾传播期预防服药?

疟疾发病有一定的地域性和规律性，因此，当地卫生防疫人员会划定一定区域分别在 8、9、10 月份服用一次磷酸哌喹，进行预防性服药，请广大群众，在当地卫生人员的指导下，配合做好疟疾的预防服药。只有得到你的合作，你和家人及周围人群才能不会得疟疾，才能阻止疟疾的传播。

-8-

四、得了疟疾怎么办?

如果你有发冷、发热，并间歇发作，有可能感染了疟疾，请赶快到村卫生室进行就诊，可免费获得疟疾治疗的药品（磷酸氯喹片/磷酸伯氨喹片组合包装），请在医生的指导下全程服完药物，如自觉病好了，中断服药会造成疟疾复发。同时做到不露宿，睡帐里，避免蚊子叮咬，将疟疾传给你的家人。

五、预防服药有哪些注意事项?

（一）应按规定剂量服药，并尽量在饭后服用。

（二）1 周岁以内、孕产妇、哺乳期妇女、年老体衰者、长期患有心血管疾病及肝肾功能不全者不宜服药。

六、服药后可能出现哪些副反应?

本药副反应较小，个别人可能出现头昏、头痛、嗜睡、乏力、恶心、呕吐、腹胀、腹泻、腹痛等，有的可能发生脸部或手足麻木感，一般会很快自行消失。极少数病例可能出现心悸、胸闷和气急等较重反应，当出现严重反应时，请与当地村医联系。

疟疾防治咨询电话：

×××疾病预防控制中心

经宣传，本人对疟疾防治基本知识已了解，并同意预防服药。

__________（签名）

年 月 日

-9-

Fig. 4.6 (**a**) Health education prescription allocated to each administration subject. (**b**) Health education prescription on the wall of a villager's home

inquiries, and other methods can help increase the medication administration rate. Each county-level government department and health department had established supervision teams, and each supervision team was responsible for its own work. Supervision by higher-level government departments is very important for ensuring the efficacy of the work at lower levels. For example, the head of Guoyang County in charge of health supervised at the township and village level for more than 10 working days during MDA each year. Bureau-level cadres were responsible for daily summary reports and progress briefings during the medication administration period. Supervisors must pay attention to methods. For example, when confirming whether drugs have been taken, one may initially ask, "How many pills are left at home?," "How many pills did you take this year?," "What color were the drugs?," and "How many days have you been taking medication?" In this supervision process, problems, such as replacing personnel on the medication delivery team and ensuring project quality, were discovered and resolved in a timely manner. At the same time, provincial-level and municipal-level staff were arranged for supervision. The Provincial Department of Health and the Provincial Center for Disease Control and Prevention organized numerous resident supervisors and multiple touring supervision teams to inspect and supervise the implementation of projects in each county. The inspection results at the end of each year's work were reported at the provincial level.

Question and Answer

18. Are there any other factors contributing to the success of MDA?

Answer:

Collecting basic data and generating an overview of all malaria cases

Before the implementation of MDA, it is necessary to obtain accurate numbers of malaria cases and people. In reality, some cases may not be detected. The reasons for this are as follows: First, some doctors may not have a sufficient understanding of the symptoms of the disease, or due to insufficient staining time and concentration of blood slides before microscopic examination, malaria parasites in the blood may not be detected, which can lead to missed diagnoses. Second, some cases are confirmed but not registered. Third, some patients do not seek medical attention. Therefore, before the implementation of MDA, it is necessary to first collect a list of all malaria cases and suspected malaria cases from local medical institutions and then conduct a detailed investigation at residents' homes to obtain a list of all cases in the area.

4.3 Part 3. Effects of MDA on the Control of *P. vivax* Malaria

From 2007 to 2014, Anhui Province had 5.951 million people participating in MDA, including 4.185 million people before the start of the transmission season and 1.766 million people during the transmission season. At the same time, standardized treatment was carried out for cases, and some mosquito vector control measures were implemented (Xia et al. 2014). The malaria burden in the province declined rapidly

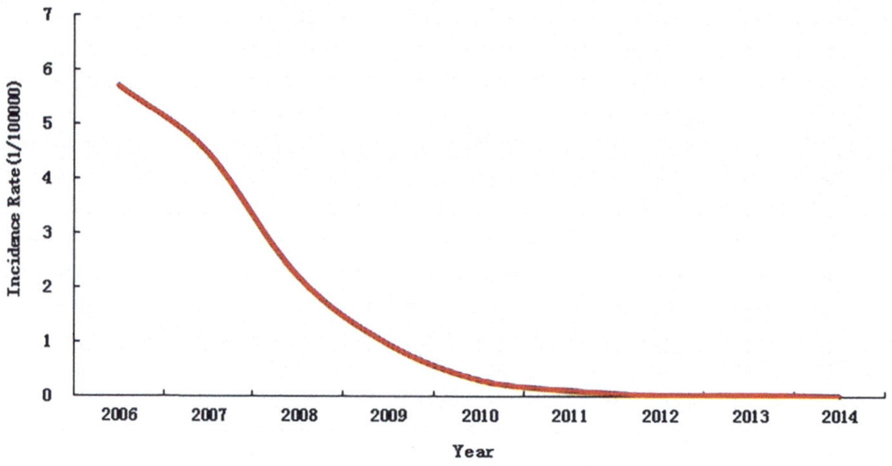

Fig. 4.7 The incidence of malaria in Anhui Province from 2006 to 2014

(Xu et al. 2015), and the reported incidence rate decreased from 57.2/100,000 people in 2006 to no local malaria cases since 2014 (Fig. 4.7).

4.4 Conclusions

The following considerations are necessary to ensure the effectiveness of MDA against *P. vivax* malaria:

1. The medication coverage area needs to be determined according to the characteristics of the malaria parasitic strain.
2. The proper drugs need to be selected according to the antimalarial mechanism of the drug and its half-life.
3. The DOT method ensures medication coverage, compliance, and safety.
4. Government leadership, extensive community participation, and the promotion of a positive atmosphere are necessary conditions for the implementation of MDA.
5. Collecting basic data and providing an overview of all malaria cases are indispensable factors behind the success of an MDA program.
6. Understanding the distribution of the population taking medication is necessary.
7. Key populations must be selected.
8. Different health education products should be tailored to the characteristics of the population.
9. Each medication recipient must receive relevant information, and informed consent must be obtained before the medication is administered.

Acknowledgments This work was supported by the Bill & Melinda Gates Foundation (No. INV-018913).

References

Gou JB, Feng ZJ, Li HZ, Zheng CJ, Ge J, Zhu G, You FH, Zhu DS (2008) Analysis of side effects caused by piperaquine phosphate for malaria prophylaxis in population. China Trop Med 4:541–543

Xia ZG, Xu JF, Zhang SS, Wang RB, Qian YJ, Zhou SS, Yang WZ, Zhou XN (2014) Determination of key interventions for the transition from control to elimination of malaria in China. Zhongguo Xue Xi Chong Bing Fang Zhi Za Zhi 6:598–601

Xu XF, Zhang XZH (2022) Anhui statistical yearbook-2022. China Statistics Press, Beijing. http://tjj.ah.gov.cn/oldfiles/tjj/tjjweb/tjnj/2022/index.htm

Xu X, Li WD, Jiang JJ, Zhang T, Wang JJ (2015) Analysis of malaria epidemic characteristics in Anhui province during 1999-2013. Chin J Parasitol Parasit Dis 33:1–6

Xu X, Zhang T, Jiang JJ, Li WD (2020) Course of malaria control and elimination in Anhui Province. J Trop Dis Parasitol 18(65–69):80

Xu X, Wang JJ, Jiang JJ, Zhang T, Lv XF, Wang SQ, Liu ZJ, Li WD, Lu XC (2022) Mass drug administration in response to vivax malaria resurgence in Anhui Province of Huanghuai plain. China Adv Parasitol 116:115–152. Epub 2022 May 31. https://doi.org/10.1016/bs.apar.2022.04.001

Zhou SS, Wang Y, Tang LH (2007) National malaria situation in 2006. Chin J Parasitol Parasit Dis 25:439–441

5.1 Retrospective Study of Malaria in Yongcheng County

On August 9, 2006, there were nine cases of malaria in Hezhuang village, Maqiao township, Yongcheng County. The staff of the local CDC were very nervous and decided to visit the village to conduct a field investigation (Fig. 5.1).

Note: Please remember the nine cases, as this is how the outbreak began

5.1.1 Part 1. Background

Yongcheng County is located on the Huanghuai Plain, where malaria transmission used to be unstable and epidemic. Historically, most malaria reemergences occurred along the Huai River in Central China. The county borders Anhui Province in the south, east, and north and goes deep into the hinterland of Anhui Province. It is known as the "gateway of eastern Henan." Administratively, the county comprises 29 townships and 737 administrative villages (the smallest administrative unit in China). The population is 1.64 million, with a density of 677 people per square kilometer. The county has five second-level hospitals, 35 health centers, and 925 health posts. Although the health facilities above health centers are government-owned, all the institutions have facilitated malaria laboratory diagnosis and treatment capabilities.

This region is a plain, with altitudes generally 31.9 m above the sea. The climate is temperate, cold in winter and hot in summer, with temperatures averaging approximately 14 °C to 15 °C throughout the year. The annual average rainfall is 874 mm, but more than two-thirds of rain falls between June and September.

Therefore, malaria is seasonal, and the starting time of malaria transmission coincides approximately with the beginning of the rainy season. The incidence of malaria in 1970 was as high as 33.68% (Zhou et al. 2009). After comprehensive prevention and control measures, the malaria prevalence declined considerably, and

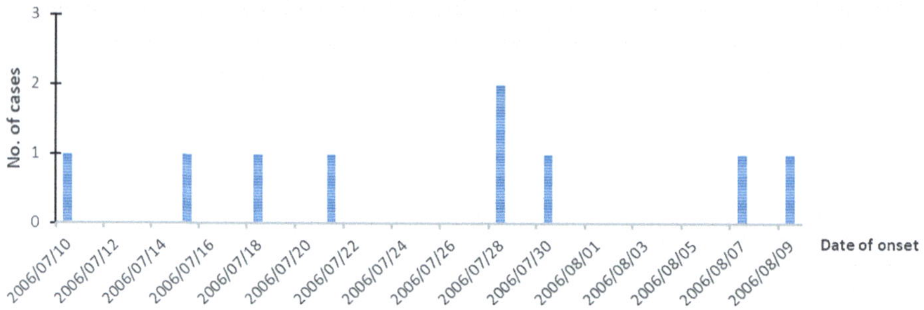

Fig. 5.1 Nine malaria cases were reported in Hezhuang village, Maqiao township, Yongcheng County from July 10 to August 9, 2006

the annual incidence rate stabilized below 1/10,000 people. No indigenous malaria cases were reported from 1992 to 2002 (Fig. 5.2).

The main malaria vector in this area is *An. sinensis.* This mosquito species has a preference for consuming cattle blood and its habit of resting outdoors has been reported in Henan Province (Zhang et al. 2019). There are obvious seasonal fluctuations for mosquito distribution, which start in late May, peak in July and August, begin to decline in late September, and disappear in November. The peak of mosquito activity is 1 h before sunset and around midnight. The larvae can be captured in the water in ponds, ditches, and subsidence areas.

Since 2003, malaria cases have dramatically increased in Yongcheng County, and 12 cases were reported in that year. In 2004 and 2005, the number of malaria cases increased by a large margin: 168 and 710 cases were reported, respectively, corresponding to 13-fold and 3.23-fold increases (Zhou et al. 2009), respectively, compared with the previous year. This upward trend in malaria cases was also observed in the surrounding areas.

For the whole province, 2304 malaria cases were reported in 2005, of which 2296 were indigenous, and 8 were imported from other areas. At the national level, there were 32,726 indigenous cases, most of which were caused by *P. vivax*.

Question and Answer

1. What is the malaria situation in your country?

Reference answer:

- Open-ended question; for example, in South Africa, the situation is…

Recommended discussion time:

- 5 min

Note: Why were CDC staff members nervous about the nine cases? (Fig. 5.3).

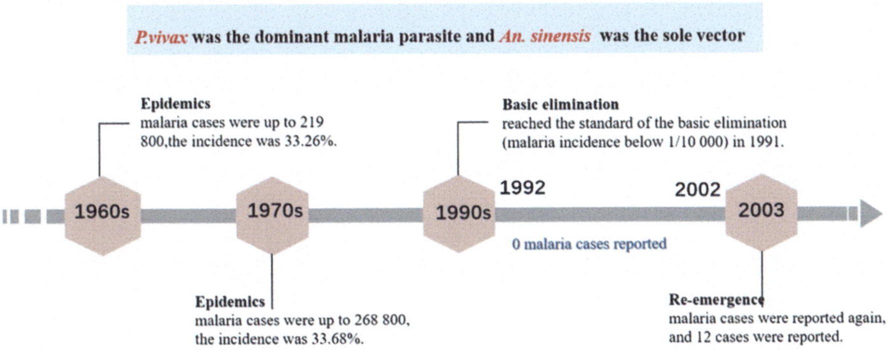

Fig. 5.2 Malaria prevalence in Henan Province

卫生部关于印发《疟疾突发疫情应急处理预案》的通知

卫疾控发[2006]第 55 号

2006 年 2 月 13 日

各省、自治区、直辖市卫生厅局，新疆生产建设兵团卫生局，各有关单位：

《疟疾暴发疫情应急处理预案《试行)》印发 2 年来，对于规范各地疟疾突发疫情应急处理和防控工作起到了积极作用。为了更好地贯彻落实《中华人民共和国传染病防治法》和《国家突发公共卫生事件应急预案》，结合各地在预案试行期间发现的问题，我部在广泛征求各省和专家意见的基础上，对预案进行了修订。现将修订后的《疟疾突发疫情应急处理预案》印发给你们，请结合本地实际贯彻执行。原卫生部办公厅印发的《疟疾暴发疫情应急处理预案(试行)》同时废止。

附件：疟疾突发疫情应急处理预案

2.1 突发疫情判定

凡出现以下情况之一时，视为疟疾突发疫情，应启动应急处理工作：

2.1.1 近 3 年无疟疾病例发生的乡（镇），1 个月内同一行政村发现 5 例及以上当地感染的疟疾病例，或发现输入性恶性疟继发病例；

2.1.2 近 3 年有疟疾病例发生的乡（镇），1 个月内同一行政村发现 10 例及以上当地感染的疟疾病例，或发现 2 例及以上恶性疟死亡病例。

2.3 突发疫情分级

I 级：在 2 个及以上相邻省份的毗邻地区出现 10 起及以上突发疫情，疫情波及 2 个及以上市(地、州），且有大范围蔓延趋势。

II 级：在 1 个省内的 2 个及以上毗邻市(地、州)出现 5 起及以上突发疫情，疫情波及 2 个及以上县(市、区)，且有扩大蔓延趋势。

III 级：在 2 个及以上毗邻的县（市、区）出现突发疫情，且有蔓延趋势。

IV 级：在 1 个县（市、区）范围内出现突发疫情。

Notice of the Ministry of Health on Issuing the 'Malaria Emergency Preparedness Plan of Action in China'

Wei Ji Kong[2006] No. 55

February 13, 2006

To the health departments and bureaus of various provinces, autonomous regions, and municipalities directly under the central government, the health bureaus of the Xinjiang Production and Construction Corps, and relevant units:

Since the publication of the 'Emergency Response Plan for Malaria Outbreaks (Trial)' two years ago, it has played a positive role in standardizing the emergency response and prevention and control of malaria outbreaks in various regions. In order to better implement the 'Law of the People's Republic of China on the Prevention and Control of Infectious Diseases' and the 'National Emergency Plan for Public Health Emergencies', combined with the problems discovered during the trial implementation of the plan in various regions, the Ministry has revised the plan on the basis of extensive consultation with provinces and experts. The revised 'Malaria Emergency Preparedness Plan of Action in China' is hereby issued to you, please implement it in conjunction with local conditions. The 'Emergency Response Plan for Malaria Outbreak (Trial)' issued by the former General Office of the Ministry of Health shall be abolished simultaneously.

Attachment: Malaria Emergency Preparedness Plan of Action in China

2.1 Determination of outbreak

Any of the following situations shall be considered as a sudden outbreak of malaria and emergency response work shall be initiated:

2.1.1 In townships/towns where there have been no malaria cases in the past three years, 5 or more locally infected malaria cases or imported secondary cases of *falciparum* malaria have been found in the same administrative village within one month;

2.1.2 In townships /towns where malaria cases have occurred in the past three years, 10 or more locally infected malaria cases or 2 or more deaths from *falciparum* malaria have been found in the same administrative village within one month.

2.3 Classification of outbreaks

Level I: There have been 10 or more outbreaks in adjacent areas of 2 or more neighboring provinces, affecting 2 or more cities/prefectures/states and showing a trend of widespread spread.

Level II: There have been 5 or more outbreaks in 2 or more adjacent cities/prefectures/states within a province, affecting 2 or more counties/cities/districts and showing a trend of expansion.

Level III: A outbreak of the epidemic has occurred in 2 or more adjacent counties/cities/districts, and there is a trend of spread.

Level IV: A sudden outbreak occurs within one county/city/district.

Fig. 5.3 Malaria Emergency Preparedness Plan of Action in China. (The content here is taken from the Malaria Control Manual in China)

According to the requirements of the Malaria Emergency Preparedness Plan of Action in China, if 10 or more indigenous cases of malaria are found in the same administrative village within a month, they should be reported as public health emergencies, and the emergency response activities should be implemented.

Question and Answer

2. Is this similar to the situation in your country? What is the threshold for initiating malaria emergency response activities in your country?

Reference answer:

- Open-ended question; for example, in my country, the situation is…

Recommended discussion time:

- 5 min

5.1.2 *Part 2. Response*

Question and Answer

3. The area was on the verge of a malaria outbreak. If you were the field epidemiological investigator, what would you do?

Reference answer:

- Open-ended question; for example, field survey, underreporting investigation, malaria vector investigation, and risk factor analysis.

Recommended discussion time:

- 5 min

5.1.2.1 Underreporting Investigation (Table 5.1)

To understand the malaria prevalence of the area, CDC staff and local village health workers conducted underreporting investigations together. As a result, 4668 residents from 956 households were investigated, and 20 malaria cases were detected. Among them, one person in a household failed to report, and the missing report rate was 8.33%. Moreover, 22 positive and 50 negative blood smears were sampled at the Maqiao health center. Therefore, the positive accordance rate was 100%, while the missed detection rate was 2% (Zhou et al. 2009).

5.1.2.2 Descriptive Epidemiology (Fig. 5.4)

From January 1 to August 15, 2006, 417 malaria cases were reported in Yongcheng County, a 2.16-fold increase over the same period of the previous year. The patients were distributed in 223 administrative villages of 28 townships, and the number of cases showed an overall tendency to increase from north to south. The highest incidence was recorded in the southern region of Yongcheng bordering northern Anhui Province. The top seven townships were Maqiao, Lizhai, Xinqia, Gaozhuang, Huangkou, Peiqiao, and Shuangqiao, accounting for 69.78% of the 417 cases reported.

Table 5.1 Underreporting investigation in Hezhuang, Yanmiao, and Panglou villages

Village	No. of cases	Visit no. of people	Screening no. of patients	No. of missing report	Missing report (%)
Hezhuang	11	1973	12	1	8.33
Yanmiao	6	1843	6	0	0
Panglou	2	852	2	0	0

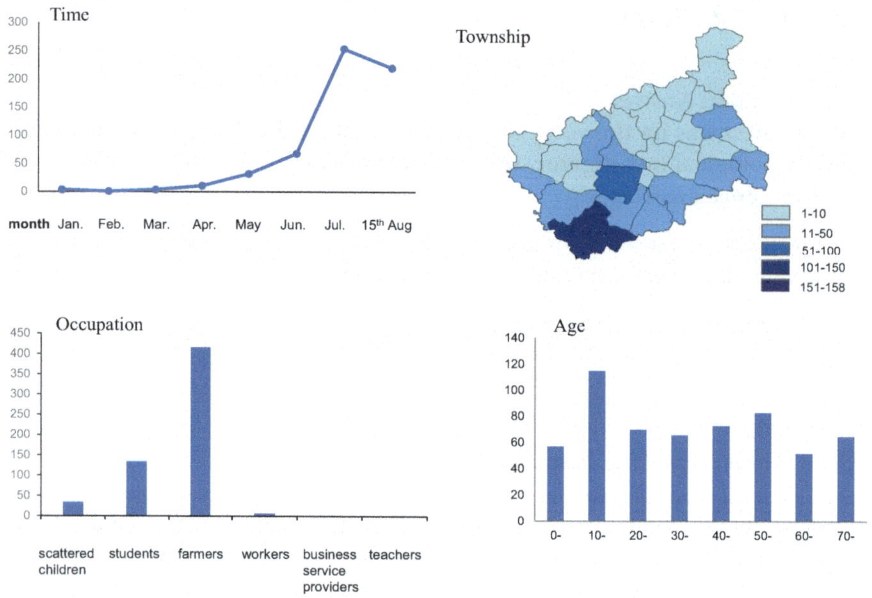

Fig. 5.4 Descriptive epidemiology in Yongcheng County

5.1.2.3 Meteorological Survey

Climatic factors, including the average monthly temperature and precipitation, were collected from January 1, 2002 to August 11, 2006. As Fig. 5.5 shows, the temperature in 2006 was above the average temperature from 2002 to 2005. The precipitation increased tremendously in June 2006. Further analysis revealed that the rainfall reached 99.6 mm on June 28. Thus, malaria cases reached a high number around August 1, approximately 30 days after the heavy rainfall.

5.1.2.4 Entomological Assessment

A total of 28 *An. sinensis* mosquitoes were captured inside houses and courtyards, all of them engorged with blood. Ring precipitation tests showed that the human blood index in Yongcheng County was 0.64 (18/28) (Pan et al. 2012).

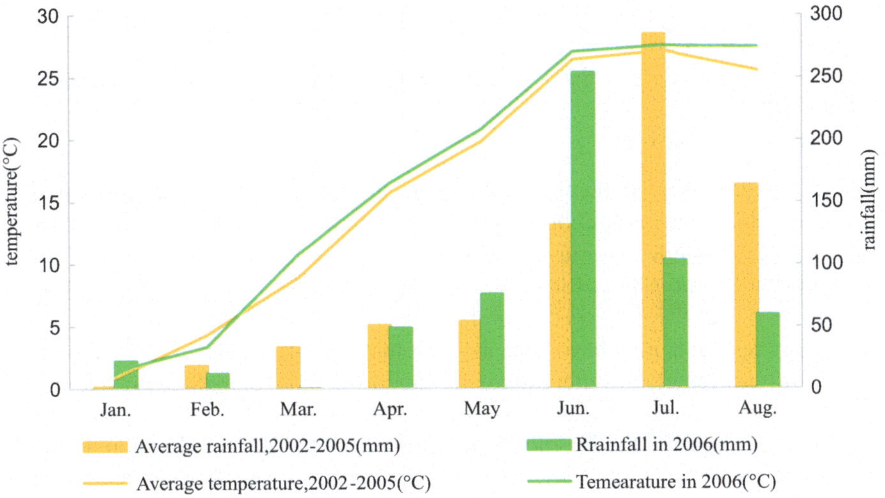

Fig. 5.5 The rainfall and temperature in 2002–2006

5.1.2.5 Field Investigation

The main crops in these areas are wheat and corn, and chemical compounds are rarely used as insecticides.

The Bao River runs through Maqiao township, and as was observed, there were also multiple open waterbodies around villages, such as gullies and small streams. Furthermore, the subsidence area of the coal mine also served as a reservoir for stagnant water. These slow-flowing, clear, and partially shaded waters are suitable habitats for *An. sinensis*, and mosquito larvae could be found in those water bodies.

A total of 7060 residents from 1614 households in affected villages were randomly selected and visited. There were 3400 mosquito nets in total, and the average number of nets per home was 2.11. Among all household members, the number of people using mosquito nets was 5499, with a proportion of 77.89%.

Residents in this area live in tile-roofed houses, which only have a front window, and most houses have screening curtains on doors and windows. However, people have a habit of being outdoors from sunset to approximately 10 p.m. Furthermore, 5.58% of household residents preferred sleeping outside during summer.

Question and Answer

4. What factors do you think possibly caused the resurgence of malaria in the area?

Reference answer:

- The Yongcheng prefecture faced strong pressure regarding the imported cases from the neighboring province. The county was surrounded by malaria-endemic counties in Anhui Province and lacked natural barriers to prevent transmission of malaria.
- *P. vivax* was the only species in the county. With its unique characteristics, many residents may have been asymptomatic. Thus, the level of *P. vivax* is always extremely low that caused the underestimation of malaria prevalence.
- Since no domestic malaria cases have been reported for 11 consecutive years, it appears that diagnosis and treatment were not timely enough due to changes in health staff, lack of microscopists, and lack of diagnosis awareness. Delays in diagnosis and treatment may negatively impact health outcomes, such as accumulation of residual loci and reintroduction of malaria.
- The overall awareness rate of malaria was low among the residents. The high temperatures during the transmission season allowed most of them to sleep and work outdoors without effective protection. This local habit accelerated the spread of malaria.
- The numerous waterbodies found around the county, including rivers, puddles, and small closed waterbodies formed by coal mining collapse, are breeding sites for *An. sinensis*.
- More precipitation with increased temperature might also contribute to malaria transmission in this area, as rainfall leads to puddles and increased humidity. These temperature increases improve the survival chances of mosquitoes.

With the progress of agricultural mechanization, fewer cattle, sheep, and pigs are raised in most areas, and as the biological barriers gradually disappear, *An. sinensis* mosquitoes may resort to biting humans.

Note: Insufficient microscopic examination capacity + increased human mosquito contact + weak net function + weak management capacity + insufficient team capacity led to the accumulation of infectious sources (core problem), followed by the increase in malaria incidence and the expansion of the epidemic scope.

Recommended discussion time:

- 8 min

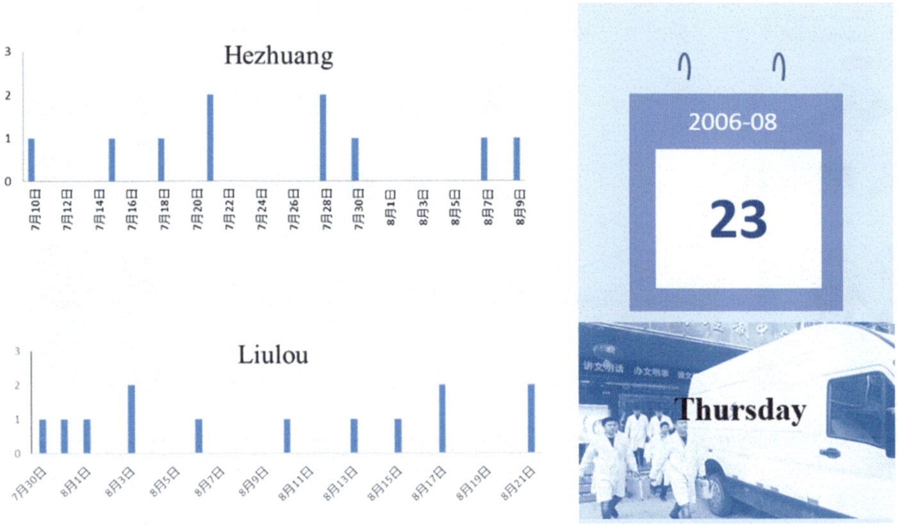

Fig. 5.6 Malaria cases in Hezhuang and Liulou villages

On August 23, 2006, 10 and 11 malaria cases were reported in Hezhuang village and Liulou village of Maqiao township, Yongcheng County, respectively. According to the requirements of the emergency response plan for malaria outbreaks issued by the Ministry of Health, the Yongcheng municipal people's government launched the emergency response plan for class IV malaria outbreaks in a timely manner (Fig. 5.6).

Question and Answer

5. What are the common control measures to deal with malaria outbreaks?

Reference answer:

Consider the three links of infectious diseases including: the source of infection, malaria vector, and the susceptible population (Fig. 5.7).

Interventions implemented (Liu et al. 2022)

1. **Strengthened case treatment and management:** Local CDC staff gave top priority to the early detection and standardized treatment of malaria cases. By distributing antimalarial drugs to village doctors, this ensured that every malaria patient received timely treatment at an early stage. Village doctors were required to deliver drugs to patients and supervise them to take the drugs daily, which ensured that every malaria patient received regular treatment.
2. **Health promotion and community participation:** Under the guidance of the Health Administrative Department, health education on malaria pre-

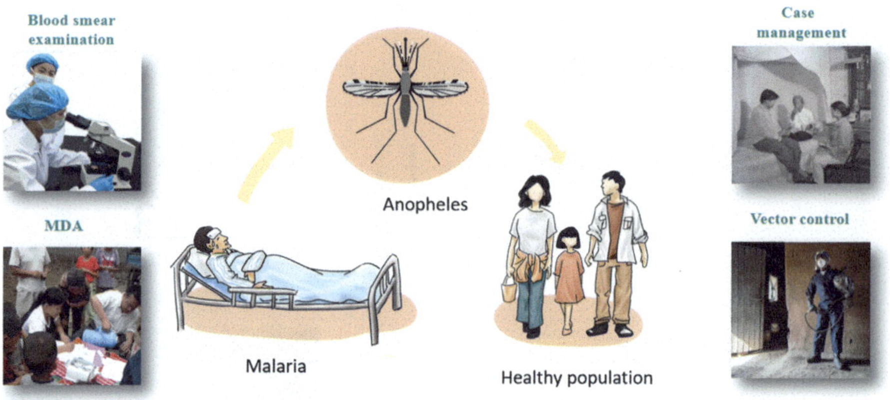

Fig. 5.7 Malaria transmission process and intervention measures. (The design and painting of these pictures were completed by Henan CDC)

vention and control information were provided to local residents through various materials such as leaflets, slogans, and billboards. Moreover, publicity calendars, brochures, and malaria information cards were distributed to residents door-to-door to improve knowledge of malaria prevention, diagnosis and treatment in this high-risk population.

3. **Vector control:** Vector control is a critical part of malaria prevention and control strategies, as it is highly effective in providing individual protection and reducing disease transmission. In addition to indoor residual spraying, bacterial larvicide control measures were implemented in 31 administrative villages where malaria outbreaks occurred in 2006.
4. **Strengthening training:** The training and retraining of technicians at county/township levels ensured and improved the capacity of malaria control measures, and the malaria-related training of village doctors ensured the timely diagnosis and standardized treatment of malaria cases.

Note: the above paragraphs focused on the measures for patients. Now let us introduce the vector control measures.

Recommended discussion time:

- 5 min

Question and Answer

6. Do you know what vector control is?

Reference answer:

- Vector control is based on vector ecology combined with social and economic development and is based on the principles of economy, safety, and not causing harm to the environment; it adopts environmental, chemical, biological and other comprehensive control measures to reduce vector population size and longevity to achieve the goal of malaria control in accordance with the location, time, and species of vector at different stages of the vector life cycle.

Recommended discussion time:

- 1 min

Question and Answer

7. Do you know anything about the *Anopheles* malaria vector?

Reference answer:

- Malaria is transmitted by the bite of female *Anopheles* mosquitoes (anophelines). The mosquito life cycle has four stages: egg, larva, pupa, and adult. The first three stages are aquatic and typically last 5–14 days, while adults can live for up to 1 month but generally for 7–14 days (WHO 2013) (Fig. 5.8).
- Anopheline larvae appear in diverse habitats worldwide, such as rice fields, puddles, ditches, and the edges of streams and rivers, but generally prefer to avoid highly polluted water. Moreover, mosquitoes generally have very different biting and resting habits, and these aspects need to be understood when making malaria vector control decisions (WHO 2013) (Fig. 5.9).

Recommended discussion time:

- 3 min

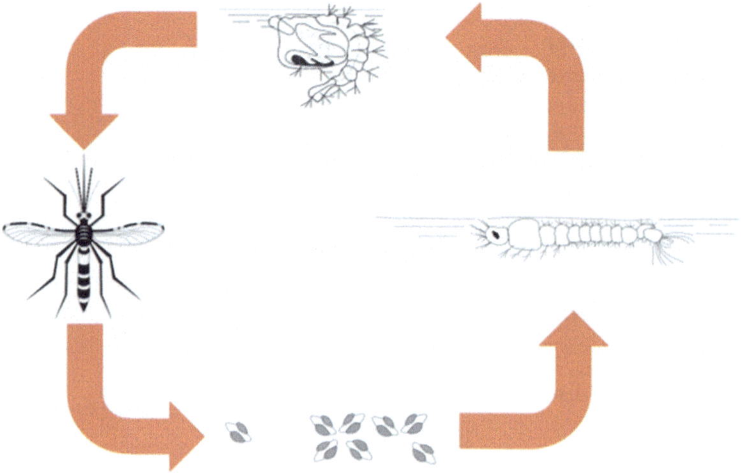

Fig. 5.8 The life cycle of anopheline mosquitoes. (The design and painting of this picture were completed by Henan CDC)

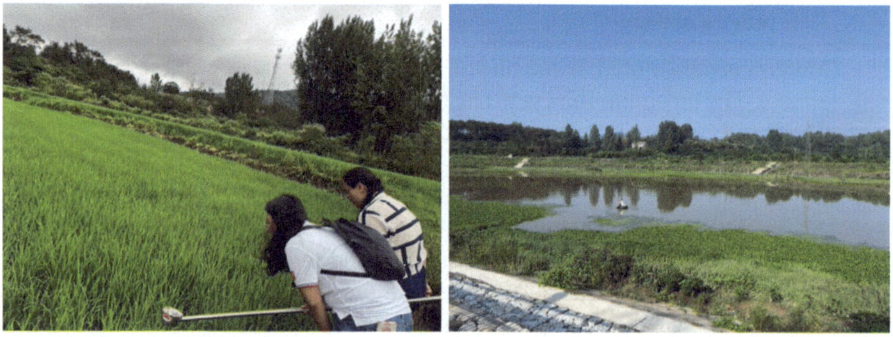

Fig. 5.9 Larval habitats. (These photos were taken by Dan Wang)

Question and Answer

8. What are the types of vector control, and how are they chosen?

Reference answer:

The WHO classifies vector control measures into four types:

Core interventions:

The recent reduction in the global burden of malaria has been largely achieved through the expansion of vector control interventions, particularly the use of insecticides for treating mosquito nets, such as long-lasting insecticidal nets (LLINs) and insecticide-treated nets (ITNs), as well as for indoor residual spraying (IRS). It is recommended to adopt core interventions (ITNs or IRS) for effective vector control in most epidemiological and ecological environments for all populations at risk of malaria (WHO 2019).

Supplementary interventions:

Complementary interventions refer to larval source management (LSM). LSM is the management of aquatic habitats that are potential larval habitats for mosquitoes to prevent the completion of immature development. Unlike LLINs and IRS, which target the adult mosquito vector, LSM targets the immature, aquatic stages (the larvae and pupae) of the mosquito, ultimately reducing the abundance of adult vectors (WHO 2013). LSM includes habitat modification and manipulation (environmental management) and larviciding.

Note: Once high coverage of core interventions has been achieved, supplementary interventions with public health value can be adopted in specific circumstances and settings (WHO 2019).

Personal protection measures

Other interventions

Vector control measures in China

Environmental governance:

Rice field irrigation system management, vegetation control, personal protection, animal barriers, and improvement of living conditions and habits are examples of environmental governance.

Chemical control:

Natural or synthetic toxic substances are used to trap, poison, and disperse mosquitoes in different ways.

Biological control:

This refers to the direct or indirect use of natural enemies or metabolites of natural enemies to control pests, mainly including catching food, parasites, and pathogens (such as bacteria) (Table 5.2).

Selection principles (WHO 2013):

1. Efficacy: Whether the intervention will reduce adult vector populations and alleviate the local transmission and impact of malaria.
2. Effectiveness: Whether the effect of the pilot stage can still be seen in ongoing activities.
3. Cost: Including costs for labor, products, monitoring and evaluation.
4. Cost-effectiveness: Whether the intervention contributes more to reducing malaria transmission than other interventions such as IRS and LLINs by less costs.
5. Environmental impact: Whether there will be any impact on the environment.
6. Safety: Ensuring the health safety of workers and communities.

Note: In view of the shortcomings of chemical control, we ultimately chose biological control.

Recommended discussion time:

- 5 min

Table 5.2 The advantages and disadvantages of the three types of vector control

Type	Advantage	Disadvantage	Example
Environmental governance	Solve the problem at the root and reduce the breeding ground of mosquitoes	It takes a long time, has a large amount of work and is not easy to manage	Habitat modification and manipulation (LSM)
Chemical control	Efficient, fast, low price	It pollutes the environment and is easy to produce drag resistance, which has an impact on human health	LLINs and IRS (Core interventions); oils and surface films (Larviciding)
Biological control	Highly efficacious against malaria vectors, selective in action, do not harm non-target organisms at the recommended doses, unlikely to produce resistance and safe for humans to handle	Slower than chemical insecticides; the control effect is often affected by climatic conditions	Bacterial larvicides (Larviciding)

Question and Answer

9. What is larviciding? What are some examples?

Reference answer:

- Larviciding is the application of biological or chemical insecticides to waterbodies regularly, including bacterial larvicides, oils and surface films, spinosyns, synthetic organic chemicals, insect growth regulators, or the introduction of natural enemies (WHO 2013).
- However, from the aspects of implementation difficulty, intervention effect, monitoring difficulty, target specificity, cost, harm to the environment, and nontarget organisms, the advantages of bacterial larvicides are more obvious.

Recommended discussion time:

- 1 min

Question and Answer

10. Do you know anything about bacterial larvicides?

Reference answer:

Bacterial larvicides include products based on the insecticidal crystal proteins produced by *Bacillus thuringiensis* ssp. *israelensis* (*Bti*) and *Bacillus sphaericus* (*Bs*) (WHO 2013).

Mode of action: After being ingested by mosquito larvae, these proteins are modified by enzymes in the midgut of the larvae and then bind to specific receptors on the midgut epithelium, leading to pore formation and disruption of feeding and homeostasis (WHO 2013).

Advantages of bacterial larvicides (WHO 2013):

1. Fast implementation of operations.
2. Harmless to nontarget organisms at the recommended doses.
3. Safe for use in a variety of habitats including drinking and irrigation water.
4. Effective in areas where mosquitoes have developed resistance to synthetic chemical larvicides.

Note: It is important to use WHOPES-recommended bacterial larvicides and formulations related to specific strain numbers to ensure biological and performance equivalency.

Two types: *Bacillus thuringiensis ssp. Israelensis* (*Bti*) and *Bacillus sphaericus* (*Bs*).

It is important to note that when using a microbial larvicide, there are only strains AM65–52 for *Bti* and AM65–52 for *Bs*. Not all larvicides are equally effective, and consideration needs to be given to their stability, potency, and their duration in the water column (WHO 2013).

Advantages and disadvantages of the two types:

- *Bti* can be applied to all habitats except very polluted habitats and must be applied weekly (WHO 2013).
- *Bs* can be applied to all habitats, including very polluted habitats, and can last a long time, but it is expensive (WHO 2013) (Fig. 5.10).

Recommended discussion time:

- 5 min

WHOPES-approved larvicides are recommended, as listed at (http://www.who.int/whopes/Mosquito_Larvicides_Sept_2012.pdf) .

Bacillus thuringiensis *subsp.* israelensis *(Bti)*	**Bacillus sphaericus *(Bs)***
In all habitats, less effective in very polluted habitats (e.g. latrines);	In all habitats – including very polluted water;
Needs to be applied weekly;	Application can give an extended residual;
Cheap.	Expensive.

Fig. 5.10 The advantages and disadvantages of *Bti* and *Bs*

Question and Answer

11. What are the factors that determine whether bacterial larvicides are appropriate?

Reference answer (WHO 2013):

- Malaria epidemiology: Malaria incidence and parasite prevalence
- Existing malaria interventions: Other ongoing interventions, for example, IRS and/or LLIN coverage
- Vector bionomics: Primary and secondary vector species; adult mosquito biting and resting habits
- Larval ecology: Nature and stability of larval habitats
- Status of vector resistance
- Economics: The cost per person protected by larviciding per year.
- Health system and national malaria control program: Capacity and commitment

The areas or municipalities that consider LSM first may have the following characteristics (WHO 2013):

- Historically or currently, the relative burden of malaria is highest in areas that typically have low to moderate transmission.
- There is a reemerging problem of malaria.
- A high population density or a low population density with clearly defined, limited and accessible breeding sites.
- Presence of other vector-borne diseases.

Recommended discussion time:

- 3 min

Question and Answer

12. What else would you like to know about bacterial larvicides?

Reference answer:

- *Economics*: High costs and acceptability have been considered to restrict the large-scale application of interventions (Regis et al. 2000), but studies have indicated that the cost of bacterial larvicides ranges from US$0.44 to 2.50 per person per year (Dambach et al. 2016), which is comparable with the costs of other vector interventions (Derua et al. 2019; USAID 2007).
- *Impact on the environment*: *Bti* and *Bs* are both naturally occurring, spore-forming bacteria found in aquatic and soil environments worldwide (WHO 2013). According to their mode of action (Becker et al. 1995; Majambere et al. 2007; Worrall and Fillinger 2011), they are target specific, do not harm nontarget organisms, and can be safely used in drinking water or irrigated crops.

Recommended discussion time:

- 3 min

Question and Answer

13. Why is Yongcheng suitable for bacterial larvicides?

Reference answer:

1. Malaria epidemiology: The malaria epidemic in Yongcheng County was one of the most serious counties in Henan Province in its history. After basic elimination, there was a resurgence of malaria epidemics.
2. Demography: Yongcheng County has a high population density, so the investment of effective resources is very necessary.
3. Larval habitats: Larval habitats are well-defined and findable. The numerous waterbodies found around the county, including rivers, puddles, and small closed waterbodies formed by coal mining collapse, are breeding sites for *An. sinensis*.
4. Adult vector ecology.
   (a) *P. vivax* was a single malaria parasite and *An. sinensis* was the only vector.
   (b) *An. sinensis* mosquitoes bite outdoors, the ratios of mosquitoes that were caught indoors and outdoors were 1:5.6 (1976), 1:10.6 (1977), and 1:7 (1978), respectively.
   (c) *An. sinensis* mosquitoes were more zoophilic. In the pilot study, the human blood index (HBI) values of *An. sinensis* collected from the

habitat around the village was 0.2588 (44/170, 1975) and 0.3049 (132/433, 1978); however, in 2006, the latest results showed a human blood index of 0.64.

5. Other interventions
   (a) Mosquito net use: A total of 7060 residents from 1614 households in affected villages were randomly selected and visited. There were 3400 mosquito nets in total, and the average number of nets per home was 2.11. Among all household members, the number of people using mosquito nets was 5499, with a rate of 77.89%.
   (b) Due to the widespread distribution of *An. sinensis*, the effectiveness of indoor and outdoor residual spraying was not satisfactory, resulting in no meaningful progress in vector control work in the region.
6. Insecticide resistance: The investigation found that *An. sinensis* developed resistance to some chemical insecticides.

Recommended discussion time:

- 3 min

Question and Answer
14. What preparations should be made before implementing biological control measures?

Reference answer:

Note: Biological control measures involve a complex process that needs to be well planned (Fig. 5.11).

- *Political support*: Maintaining and securing political support for an LSM program is crucial for several reasons: (1) to increase the likelihood that governments will provide any additional funding needed for LSM in the malaria control program, (2) to facilitate collaboration between the Ministry of Health and other sectors, and 3) to facilitate the establishment of new legislation on mandatory removal of certain larval habitats or preventing the creation of new larval habitats (WHO 2013).
- *Selection of the intervention sites*: Intervention sites and untreated sites are identified based on malaria incidence.
- *Community sensitization*: The administration, community leaders, and community members must be informed and agree before any larviciding is carried out in the intervention area. Community members are usually very concerned about any pesticide applied by research teams (USAID 2007). There is usually concern that pesticides sprayed in water will affect humans or livestock.

Community sensitization can be performed in a variety of ways (WHO 2013):

- Meetings with prominent community leaders/members.
- Public addresses using a loudspeaker on a car in all the streets before the intervention.
- Distribution of frequently asked question documents and leaflets at all meetings.
- *Training field staff*: Field staff should receive training in mapping and characterizing larval habitats, finding and identifying mosquito larvae and pupae, and selecting LSM methods in the area. In addition, staff involved in larviciding should receive training in the standard operating procedures of larviciding (WHO 2013).
- *Baseline mapping and data collection*: First, the larvae habitats and waterbodies need to be mapped. Second, data on larval and adult populations must be collected, preferably over 1 year or one transmission season. This enables the identification of the main larval habitats and vector species and allows for good planning and targeting of LSM. It also helps to evaluate the impact of the intervention.

The Yongcheng leading group on bacterial Larvicides headed by the mayor-in-charge was established, which is responsible for the organization, management, command, and coordination of bacterial larvicide work. The municipal government allocated 800,000 RMB (yuan) as a special fund for the purchase of pesticides, personnel subsidies, and other expenses. This work has received strong support from the local government. Village cadres publicize malaria control knowledge in person and promote the measures through various means such as slogans and leaflets to improve the cooperation of residents. Training of field staff is also performed, including breeding site characterization and mapping, method selection, and larval instar identification.

Recommended discussion time:

- 3 min

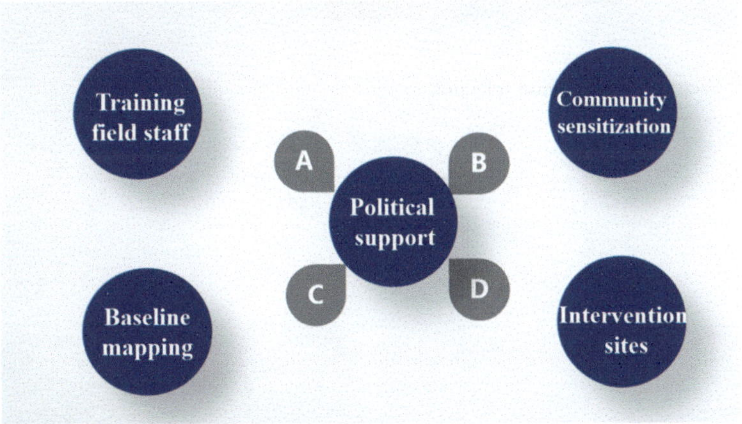

Fig. 5.11 Preparation before implementation

Question and Answer

15. Can we use bacterial larvicides?

Reference answer:

Selection of biological agents: WHOPES-approved larvicides are recommended.

Bacillus thuringiensis ssp. *israelensis* (*Bti*)

Bacillus sphaericus (*Bs*)

Formulations: Larvicides are generally available as granules, water-dispersible granules (WGs), wettable powders (WPs), suspension concentrates (SCs), and briquettes (BRs). Biological activity is expressed in international toxic units per milligram (ITU/mg) (WHO 2013) (Fig. 5.12).

Equipment: The selection of equipment, equipment calibration, and training of application personnel are crucial to the success of the operations. The types of sprayers can be selected according to the available equipment, habitat types, and specific application targets (WHO 2013) (Fig. 5.13).

Recommended discussion time:

- 3 min

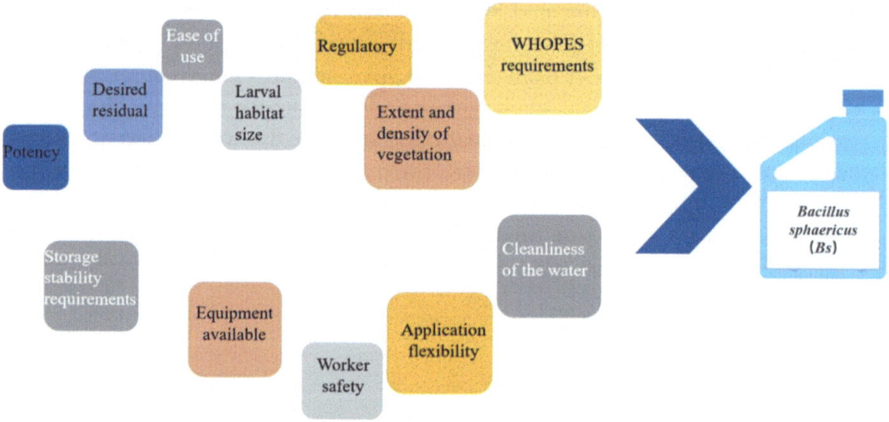

Fig. 5.12 Factors in formulation selection

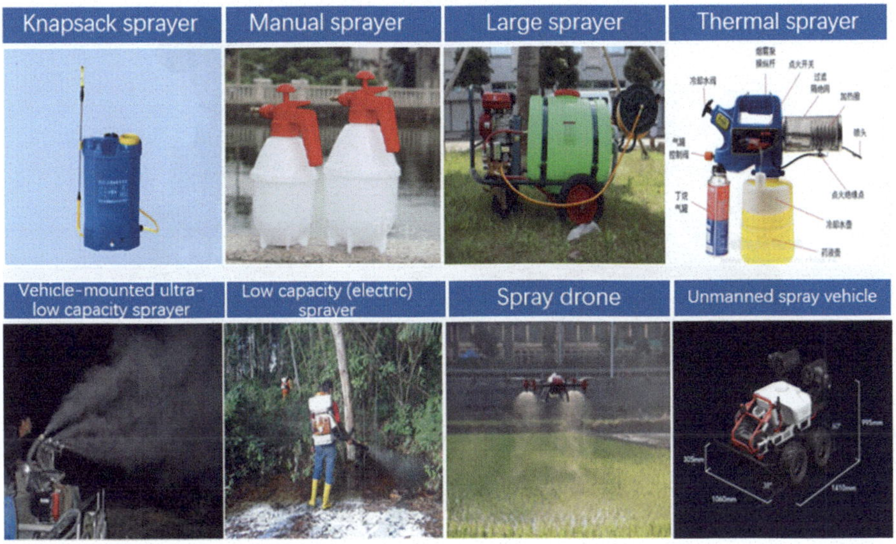

Fig. 5.13 Types of sprayers. (Reprinted with permission from Springer Nature)

Question and Answer

16. How are bacterial larvicides applied?

Reference answer:

- From August 20 to the end of October 2006, 31 administrative villages with malaria outbreaks were selected to implement bacterial larvicide control measures. All breeding sites in those villages were covered with larvicides, regardless of water depth. In addition, 8 mL/m^2 suspending agent of the commercial strains of *Bacillus sphaericus* (*Bs.*) (Lvyuan Biochemical Co., Ltd., Yangzhou, Jiangsu, China, 100 ITU/mg) were nebulized by electric sprayers (Hudson 1035BP, diameter $\leq$ 50 μm) at intervals of 15 days for 2 months. The treatment concentrations were described in a previous study (Figs. 5.14 and 5.15).

Recommended discussion time:

- 3 min

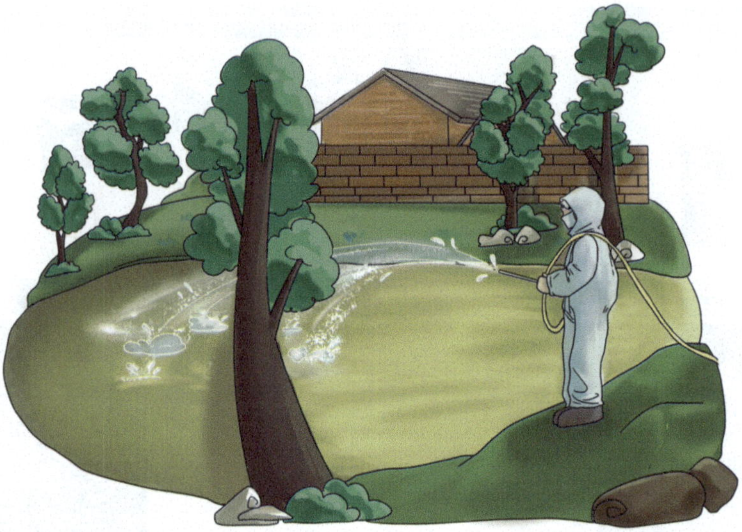

Fig. 5.14 Thirty-one administrative villages were selected to carry out biological mosquito control measures from August 20 to the end of October 2006. (The design and drawing of this picture were completed by Henan CDC staff)

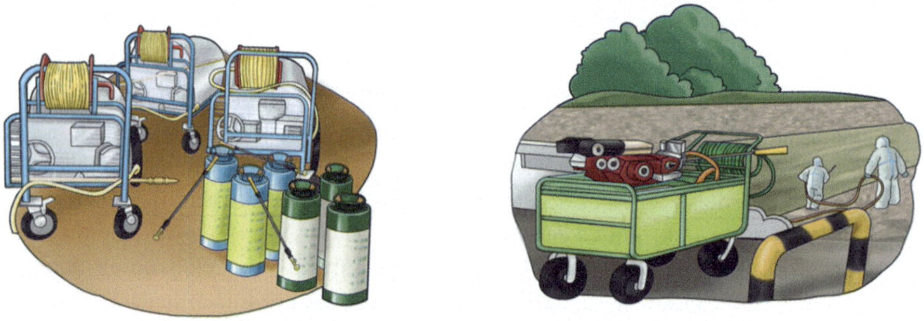

Production provider: Jiangsu Yangzhou Lvyuan Biochemical Co., Ltd

Dosage: 8 ml / m^2 (surface of the water)

Specification: SC, 100 ITU mg

Sprayer: Hsun 1035 BP type (grain diameter less than 50 μm)

Frequency: once every 15 days

Fig. 5.15 Bacterial larvicides were delievered in Yongcheng County. (The design and painting of these pictures were completed by Henan CDC staff)

5.1.3 Part 3. Evaluation

Monitoring and evaluation are integral parts of the vector control program to document progress toward the objectives and to make data-driven decisions at all levels of the program (WHO 2013). It is necessary to monitor whether the larvicide is effective and whether there are substantial reductions in larvae and adult vector densities compared to baseline.

To assess the impact of larviciding, both larval and adult surveillance were undertaken regularly. Throughout the study period, eight larval habitats from the treatment and control sites were randomly selected, and surveillance was performed one day prior to and one day after the intervention.

Mosquito larvae were sampled using dippers, and ten dips (500 ml) were taken per sentinel site to determine the larval density. Adult mosquito abundance was monitored by the human trap method 3 h after sunset. The percentage reduction was calculated as follows: reduction (%) = 100−(C1/T1* T2/C2) *100, where C1 and T1 indicate the density of larvae (or adults) in the control and treated habitats before treatment, respectively, whereas C2 and T2 refer to post-treatment (Fig. 5.16 and Tables 5.3 and 5.4).

After a 24-h exposure to *Bs.* strains, each stage of instar larvae of *An. sinensis* could be seen. The reduction in the larval density was up to 76.2%, while only the first instar larvae were present by the 14th day. Larval density was reduced by 100% after the fourth spraying when compared with baseline. Likewise, the density of the adult vector population decreased by 64%. However, the population increased following a sudden rainfall after the second spraying. After the penultimate and last rounds, 50% and 100% of the adult malaria vectors were killed, respectively. Such changes were not observed in the control group (Zhou et al. 2009) (Fig. 5.17 and Table 5.5).

The incidence of malaria in the treated villages decreased by 51.02% in 2007 compared to 2006. The decrease in the control villages was 40.0%. The morbidity in the treated villages was lower than that in the control villages ($p < 0.000$). The cumulative effect was also evaluated. For the whole county, there were 1590 malaria

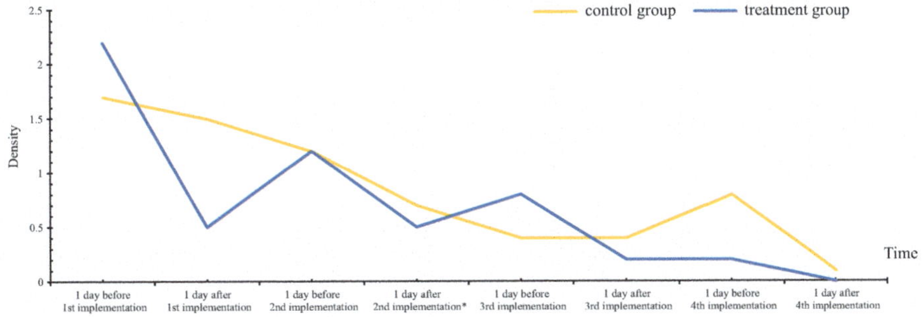

Fig. 5.16 Effect of *Bacillus sphaericus* on the density of *An. sinensis* larvae

Table 5.3 Effect of *Bacillus sphaericus* on the density of *An. sinensis* larvae

Spraying times	Control group density			Spraying group density (decline rate: %)		
	1 day before implementation	2 days after implementation	14 days after implementation	1 day before implementation	2 days after implementation	14 days after implementation
1	1.7	1.5	1.2	2.2	0.5(76.2)	1.2(24.5)
2[a]	1.2	0.7	0.4	1.2	0.5(32.4)	0.8(−9.1)
3	0.4	0.4	0.8	0.8	0.2(75.6)	0.2(85.3)
4	0.8	0.1	–	0.2	0(100)	–

[a]Rainfall on the night of drug spraying

Table 5.4 Effect of *Bacillus sphaericus* on the density of *An. sinensis* adults

Spraying times	Control group density			Spraying group density (decline rate: %)		
	1 day before implementation	2 days after implementation	14 days after implementation	1 day before implementation	2 days after implementation	14 days after implementation
1	3.0	3.0	2.0	5.5	2(63.6)	2.3(36.4)
2[a]	2.0	2.0	1.0	2.3	2(14.3)	0.7(42.9)
3	1.0	1.0	2.0	0.7	0.3(50)	0.3(75)
4	2.0	1.0	–	0.3	0(100)	–

[a]Rainfall on the night of drug spraying

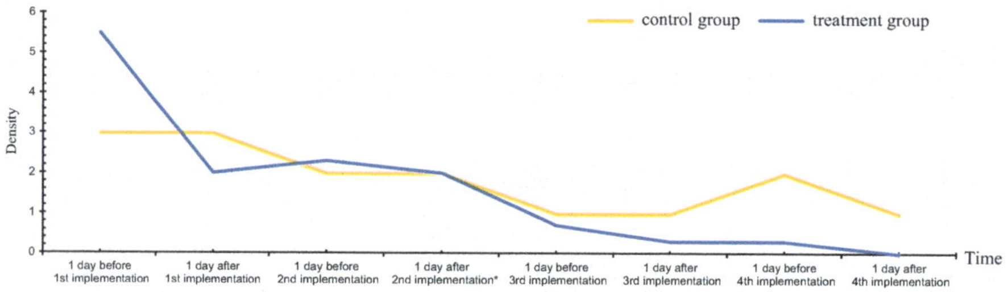

Fig. 5.17 Effect of *Bacillus sphaericus* on the density of *An. sinensis* adults

Table 5.5 The incidence rates in treatment and control villages in 2006–2007

Region	2006		2007		Increase or decrease rate (%)
	No. of cases	Incidence rate (%)	No. of cases	Incidence rate (%)	
Treatment village	663	0.98	323	0.48	−51.02
Control village	1467	0.90	885	0.54	−40.0

cases in 2007, declining from the 2890 reported in 2006. The incidence was statistically significant according to the χ^2 test (Zhou et al. 2009) ($p < 0.000$).

5.2 Application Effect of Bacterial Larvicides in Africa

Bs and *Bti* has been tested in African ecosystems with significant effectiveness in control of malaria transmission. For instance, Gambia conducted a pilot-scale field study on the floodplain of the Gambia River from August to November 2005. Liquid (WDGs) and granule (CGs) formulations of both *Bs* and *Bti* were tested. Weekly application of *Bs* resulted in 100% mortality of late instar larvae at any application date regardless of the formulation applied. Weekly application of *Bti* under operating conditions throughout the 9-week study period, regardless of the formulation and equipment used, achieved sustained suppression of larval development with minimum dosages (as determined in the laboratory) (Regis et al. 2000) (Fig. 5.18).

The Cotonou City in the Republic of Benin applied bacterial larvicides from May 2007 to July 2008. *Bti* was sprayed in all mosquito habitats in the "sprayed zone." Spraying was carried out every other week by a team of 12 operators. The incidence of clinical malaria among children under 5 years of age decreased from 37% in 2006 to 31% in 2008 in the sprayed zone, while in the nonsprayed zone, the incidence of clinical malaria increased from 33% in 2006 to 36% in 2008 (Kinde-Gazard and Baglo 2012) (Fig. 5.19).

Drawing on the large-scale community-based larviciding program conducted by the Urban Malaria Control Programme in Dar es Salaam (United Republic of Tanzania), the investigators estimated the cost-effectiveness of larviciding for

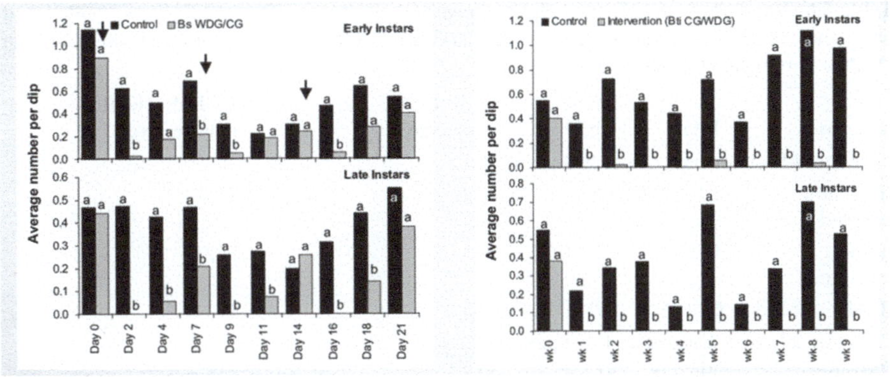

Fig. 5.18 Efficiency of *Bs* or *Bti* treatments under field-operating conditions in Gambia (Regis et al. 2000)

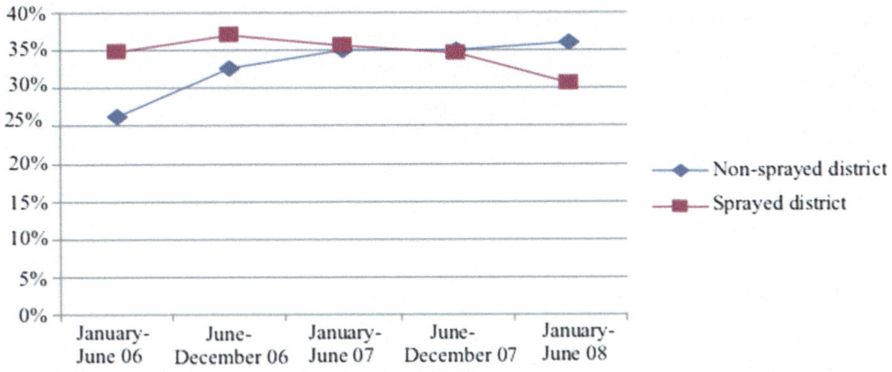

Fig. 5.19 Evaluation of malaria morbidity in the sprayed district compared to the control district in Benin (Kinde-Gazard and Baglo 2012). (Reprinted with permission from Elsevier)

malaria control in urban areas of sub-Saharan Africa (Dambach et al. 2016; Maheu-Giroux and Castro 2014).

The cost-effectiveness of larviciding has been shown to be highly dependent on the assumed baseline malaria incidence. Cost-effectiveness ratios (CERs) are reported for the following health outcomes: disability-adjusted life years (DALYs) avoided, malaria infections averted, and malaria-associated deaths prevented. The WHO states that interventions with a CER per DALY averted less than a country's per capita gross domestic product (GDP) could be regarded as "very cost-effective" and those for which the cost-effectiveness is less than three times the country's per capita GDP could be considered "cost-effective." Given Tanzania's per capita GDP of US$599 (2012), larviciding can be considered very cost-effective in various transmission scenarios (Maheu-Giroux and Castro 2014) (Table 5.6).

Table 5.6 Number of cases averted, deaths prevented, disability-adjusted life years avoided, and gross and net cost-effectiveness ratios for the larviciding intervention in Dar es Salaam, Tanzania (Maheu-Giroux and Castro 2014)

Scenarios	Total	Gross CER[a]	CER[a] Provider's perspective	**CER[a] Societal perspective**
Scenario #1—incidence rate of 902 per 1000				
Infection averted	1,178,999	$4.3	$3.6	$2.4
Death prevented	1265	$4040	$3345	$2213
DALY averted	65,125	$78.5	$65.0	$43.0
Scenario #2—incidence rate of 227 per 1000				
Infection averted	296,228	$17.3	$16.5	$15.3
Death prevented	318	$16,077	$15,383	$14,250
DALY averted	16,363	$312.4	$298.9	$276.9
Scenario #3—incidence rate of 122 per 1000				
Infection averted	159,282	$32.1	$31.3	$30.1
Death prevented	171	$29,900	$29,206	$28,073
DALY averted	8798	$580.9	$567.4	$545.4

Note: All prices are in 2012 US dollars
[a]*CER* cost-effectiveness ratio

5.2.1 Part 4. Conclusions

Bacterial larvicides can be a useful supplement to core interventions (LLINs and IRS) but only in some specific locations and need to be scaled up as a pilot based on successful practical applications.

On the basis of comprehensive prevention and control measures, bacterial larvicides were also adopted to control the outbreak of malaria in Yongcheng County.

Bacterial larvicides are an effective intervention against malaria and are expected to be applied on a large scale in Africa.

Acknowledgments This work was supported by the Bill & Melinda Gates Foundation (No. INV-018913).

References

Becker N, Zgomba M, Petric D, Beck M, Ludwig M (1995) Role of larval cadavers in recycling processes of *Bacillus sphaericus*. J Am Mosq Control Assoc 11(3):329–334

Dambach P, Schleicher M, Stahl H-C, Traoré I, Becker N, Kaiser A et al (2016) Routine implementation costs of larviciding with *bacillus thuringiensis israelensis* against malaria vectors in a district in rural Burkina Faso. Malar J 15(1):380

Derua YA, Kweka EJ, Kisinza WN, Githeko AK, Mosha FW (2019) Bacterial larvicides used for malaria vector control in sub-Saharan Africa: review of their effectiveness and operational feasibility. Parasit Vectors 12(1):426

Kinde-Gazard D, Baglo T (2012) Assessment of microbial larvicide spraying with *Bacillus thuringiensis israelensis*, for the prevention of malaria. Med Mal Infect 42(3):114–118

Liu Y, He ZQ, Wang D, Hu YB, Qian D, Yang CY, Zhou RM, Li SH, Lu DL, Zhang HW (2022) One health approach to improve the malaria elimination programme in Henan Province. Adv Parasitol 116:153–186

Maheu-Giroux M, Castro MC (2014) Cost-effectiveness of larviciding for urban malaria control in Tanzania. Malar J 13:477

Majambere S, Lindsay SW, Green C, Kandeh B, Fillinger U (2007) Microbial larvicides for malaria control in The Gambia. Malar J 6:76

Pan JY, Zhou SS, Zheng X, Huang F, Wang DQ, Shen YZ et al (2012) Vector capacity of *Anopheles sinensis* in malaria outbreak areas of Central China. Parasit Vectors 5:136

Regis L, Silva SB, Melo-Santos MAV (2000) The use of bacterial larvicides in mosquito and black fly control programmes in Brazil. Mem Inst Oswaldo Cruz 95(suppl 1):207–210

USAID (2007) Prepared for RTI International by Liverpool Associates in Tropical Health under contract to the Bureau for Global Health. USAID, Washington, DC

WHO (2013) Larval source management: a supplementary measure for malaria control 2013. An operational manual. WHO, Geneva

WHO (2019) Guidelines for malaria vector control. WHO, Geneva

Worrall E, Fillinger U (2011) Large-scale use of mosquito larval source management for malaria control in Africa: a cost analysis. Malar J 10:338

Zhang HW, Zhang QQ, Yang CY, Qian D, Lu DL, Zhao YL et al (2019) Progress of malaria elimination and achievements of scientific researches in Henan province. Henan J Prev Med 30:721–725

Zhou GC, Zhang HW, Su YP, Zhou YS, Huang F (2009) Investigation into the results of control of malaria outbreak in Yongcheng County by biological control of mosquito larvae. China Trop Med 9(02):228

Chapter 6
Discovery History of Artemisinin

Yang-Mu Huang, Yi-Nuo Sun, Guang-Qi Liu, Yu-Ming Liu, and Yan Xie

Theme
Discovery History of Artemisinin.

Target Audience
Policymakers in government or industry; related researchers.

Learning Objectives
After completion of this case study, participant should be able to

1. Learn the chronological context and historical backdrop of China's antimalarial drugs research.
2. Understand the entire process involved in China's antimalarial drugs R&D.
3. Comprehend the use of modern methods for traditional medicine development.
4. Reflect on the role of government in drug R&D under resource-constrained conditions.
5. Identify suitable directions and methodologies for domestic drug R&D.

Y.-M. Huang (✉) · Y.-N. Sun · G.-Q. Liu · Y.-M. Liu · Y. Xie
Department of Global Health, Peking University School of Public Health, Beijing, People's Republic of China

Institute for Global Health, Peking University, Beijing, People's Republic of China
e-mail: ymhuang@bjmu.edu.cn

X.-N. Zhou, J.-H. Yin (eds.), *Malaria Control and Elimination in China*,
https://doi.org/10.1007/978-981-97-8719-7_6

Overview

In the 1950s and 1960s, the global malaria eradication campaign, initiated by the World Health Organization, faced a significant obstacle with the emergence of insecticide and drug resistance. The onset of the Vietnam War underscored the need for effective medicines, recognizing the potential strategic importance of a malaria cure in the conflict. In response, the U.S. Army Research Institute (Walter Reed) initiated collaborative research with European partners to explore alternative malaria drugs. Concurrently, in response to the Vietnamese government's request, China launched the "523 project" (named after its official start date May 23, 1967), which aimed to integrate Chinese drugs and acupuncture to identify new drug treatments for fighting chloroquine-resistant malaria, develop long-term preventative measures against chloroquine-resistant malaria, and develop mosquito repellents.

During the 1960s, China's GDP per capita was $1050, lagging behind East Asia at $1607 and the global average at $4868. Aligning with global drug development standards has proven to be a daunting task due to the lack of a mature drug administration and patent system, coupled with the context of the Cold War, which complicates drug development with global standards.

Despite these obstacles, China capitalized on its rich heritage of traditional medicine and fostered collaboration among various departments. This collective effort led to the discovery of Artemisinin, a breakthrough in malaria treatment that differed from conventional Western approaches. Under the leadership of National 523 Office and the Provincial 523 Offices, research institutes, including scientific research centers, medical colleges, and pharmaceutical factories across provinces, were mobilized. Four specialized collaborative research groups were formed, each focusing on chemical synthetic medicine, traditional Chinese medicine (TCM), repellent, and on-site prevention and control.

This discovery demonstrated that integrating traditional medicine into modern methodologies not only held promise but also proved to be a time-efficient strategy for drug research and development (R&D). Collaboration at the national level proved to be crucial to advancing research. Various tasks were efficiently executed, including investigating resources, refining extraction methods, conducting pharmacological and toxicological studies, optimizing dosage forms, establishing quality standards, and determining chemical structures.

This case study presents the discovery of artemisinin in China within the constraints of limited resources and amidst a unique international context. By articulating China's experiences, this case study aims to offer valuable perspective for other developing countries, acquaint readers with essential concepts, processes, and challenges, and guide them in formulating effective strategies for their own domestic R&D of new drugs.

6.1 Part 1. Where Did We Start?

6.1.1 Information 1

In 1965, 53,492,988 km^2 of land was affected by malaria, representing 36.65% of the total global land area. The population exposed to malaria totaled 1,924,360,320, accounting for 57.21% of the global population. In 1968, Lysenko created a global malaria-epidemic map, that categorized parasite infection rates into three levels: low prevalence (<0.1), moderate prevalence (0.11–0.5), and high prevalence (0.51–0.75) (Fig. 6.1) (Hay et al. 2004) (Table 6.1).

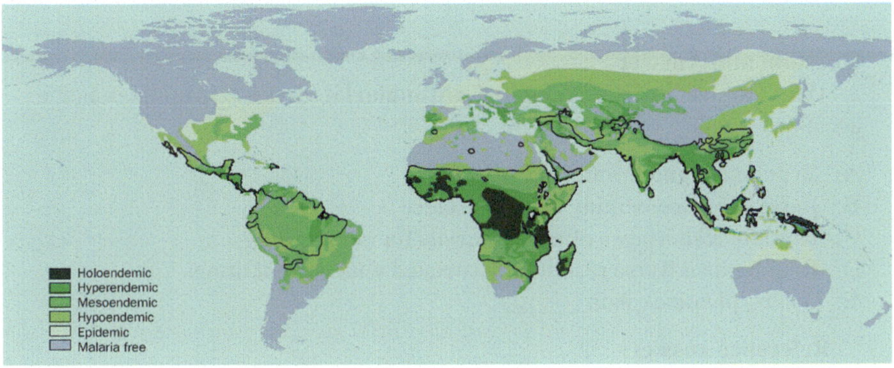

Fig. 6.1 Global malaria epidemic map in 1960s

Table 6.1 List of anti-malarial drug on record (Tse et al. 2019; Croft 2007)

Drug name	Application time	Origin	Antimalarial effect	Periods used
Cinchona bark and cinchona cream	Before the seventeenth century	Bark of cinchona tree	/	/
Quinine	Since 1820	Bark of cinchona/ artificial synthesis	Treating multiple drug-resistant plasmodium falciparum combined with tetracycline	1820–1980
Quinoline antimalarial drugs	Since 1925	Artificial synthesis	Treating malaria symptoms in the secondary erythrocytic phase; killing effect on plasmodium in the erythrocytic phase	1925–1960
Pyrimidine antimalarials	Since 1949	Artificial synthesis	Prevent malaria by acting on the primary erythrocytic phase of plasmodium	1949–
Mefloquine	/	Artificial synthesis	/	1976–1989

Question and Answer
1. Could you find your country on the global malaria-epidemic map? What was the situation at that time, and has it changed in recent times?
(As an opening question to raise interest)
Reference answer:

- For example, in Cameroon, the situation was…

Recommended discussion time:

- 6 min

Question and Answer
2. Why do we keep developing antimalarial drugs? [Multiple-choice question]

A. To pursue higher profits
B. To respond to emerging drug resistance
C. To address shortages of raw materials for current drug
D. To mitigate adverse reactions associated with current drugs
E. Others, please explain______

Reference answer:

- All choices are reasonable, but in this case, B is the right one.
- Teaching point: Drug resistance (Wernsdorfer and Kouznetsov 1980; D'Alessandro and Buttiëns 2001; Farooq and Mahajan 2004).

Resistance of human Plasmodium to modern synthetic antimalarial drugs became apparent shortly after the widespread use of these medications. Initial reports of resistance to pyrimidine and proguanidine surfaced in the early 1930s. By the early 1960s, resistance of *Plasmodium falciparum* to 4-aminoquinoline was documented in Asia and South America. The contribution of monotherapy and misuse of antimalarial drugs in contributing to the emergence of drug resistance became evident during the Global Malaria Eradication campaign initiative by the World Health Organization in 1955.
Recommended discussion time:

- 10 min

6.1.2 *Information 2*

Malaria posed a significant threat during the Vietnam War, leading to substantial depletion of military personnel on both sides. During this time, commonly used antimalarial drugs, such as chloroquine, exhibited reduced effectiveness due to antimicrobial resistance. As a result, the availability of effective antimalaria drugs became a critical determinant influencing war outcome ("523" 2015; Liu et al. 2022; Harrison and Yim 2017) (Table 6.2).

Table 6.2 China in the 1960s: Snapshot (State Statistics Bureau n.d.; Our World in Data 2021)

R&D input *GDP*	<0.56% (in 1990, China's percentage was 0.56% and the world average was 1.97%)
Research personnel *per million people*	<547.30 (in 2000, China's number was 547.30 and the world average was 1081.27)
Economy *per capita GDP*	$70 in 1962 (in 1962, the East Asian average was $146, and the world average was $482)
Malaria burden *prevalence*	0.51–0.75% in 1965 (in Southern areas of China)
Medical resources *Number of beds per 1000 people*	1.54 in 1970 (in 1970, the world average was 3.08)

Qinghao, the Chinese name of *Atremisia annua* L., has been used in China for over two millennia for its therapeutic properties in alleviating deficiency heat, hectic fever, summer heat, malaria, and jaundice (Li et al. 2017).

In China's artemisinin R&D initiative, four specialized research groups were established, aiming at chemical synthetic medicine, TCM, repellent and on-site prevention and treatment.

The TCM Group collected and screened numerous Chinese medicinal prescriptions and herbal medicine samples. They identified several herbs with effective constituents, including yingzhaosu and artemisinin.

The Chemical Synthetic Medicine Group was tasked with designing and synthesizing over 10,000 chemicals. Although several showed protective effects against malaria, none matched the impactful efficacy of artemisinin (Zhang 2015).

Question and Answer

3. What prompted China to turn to traditional medicine?

Reference answer:

- Under the political pressure from the U.S. government, the Walter Reed Army Institute of Research launched a program to find alternative antimalarial drugs. Given the scale and urgency of the task, 175 external contractors were involved in this collaborative research. More than 250,000 potential antimalarial compounds were screened and two compounds, mefloquine and halofantrine, were eventually marketed.
- China's R&D capabilities were less promising, making it challenging to undertake the massive screening of potential antimalaria compounds like America. China's extensive history of traditional medicine, spanning over 2000 years, influenced the direction of research and expedited the exploration period.

Recommended discussion time:

- 6 min

Question and Answer
4. What challenges do developing countries face in drug R&D? Are the challenges similar to your country's? [Multiple-choice question]

A. Insufficient budget
B. Shortage of research personnel
C. Challenges in conducting on-site clinical trials (e.g., literacy barriers)
D. Limited supervision and guidance
E. Others, please explain______

Reference answer:

– All choices are reasonable. New drug development requires long-term investments, multidisciplinary knowledge and technologies, and a well-established regulatory agency. All of these were weak in LMIC because of economic and social factors.

Recommended discussion time:

– 10 min

Question and Answer
5. Why was antimalarial drug R&D highly prioritized in China? Can you identify other important factors that put the issue on the government's agenda? [Single-choice question]

A. High prevalence of targeted disease
B. Public health emergency
C. Demand of wartime
D. Profit-driven motives
E. Enhancement of national impact by traditional medicine
F. Foreign aid or political needs
G. Others, please explain______

Reference answer:

– C.

Recommended discussion time:

– 10 min

6.2 Part 2. How Did We Do?

6.2.1 Information 3 (Figs. 6.2 and 6.3)

Question and Answer

6. How was the artemisinin R&D initiative organized in China? [Single-choice question]

A. Government-led
B. Researcher-led
C. Medical colleges-led
D. Pharmaceutical factory-led
E. Others, please explain______

Reference answer:

- A.
- Government-led pattern is applicable when there is a significant national development need for the drug. This approach is characterized by the government's commitment to ensuring implementation and quick mobilization of research resources.
- Researcher-led pattern and medical colleges-led pattern are suitable for advancing theoretical breakthroughs in pharmacology and can be applied to new drug development. These patterns emphasize adherence to R&D norms and foster strong innovation, with less focus on immediate drug commercialization.
- Pharmaceutical factory-led pattern is suitable for drugs with high-profit margins and where private enterprise has the necessary technology, patents and resources for development. This pattern emphasizes market considerations, patent protection, and the input–output ratio of drug development.

Recommended discussion time:

- 12 min.

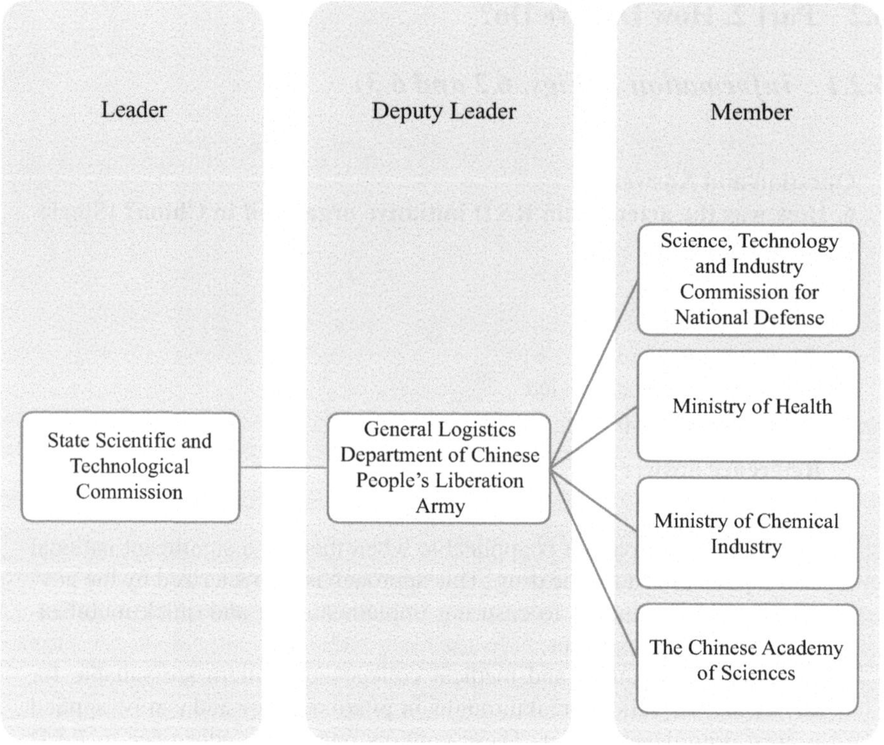

Fig. 6.2 Organization structure of national 523 office (Li et al. 2017)

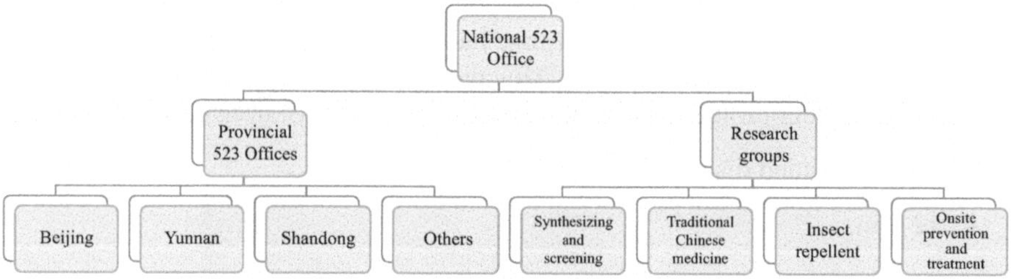

Fig. 6.3 Research responsibilities of members[8] (Li et al. 2017)

6.2.2 Information 4

Capitalizing on its extensive knowledge of TCM, China held a distinct advantage in the development of new antimalarial drugs. Chinese scientists drew inspiration from TCM books and folk recipes to screen over 40,000 herbs and compounds. Scientific research teams from Beijing, Guangdong, Guangxi, Sichuan, Yunnan, Jiangsu, and other places conducted in-depth investigations and collected folk remedies.

One notable instance occurred when the 523 Chinese herbal medicine research team in Nanjing found that in 1969, rural doctors and people in Gaoyou County, Jiangsu Province, successfully used the local Qinghao (*Artemisia annua* Linn) to treat and prevent malaria. This local wisdom was even found expressed in a folk song "Don't worry after contracting malaria, take brown sugar and Qinghao."

After consolidation of available evidence, ten herbs, including Changshan (anti-feverile dichroa root), Yingzhao (*Ar. hexapetalus*), and Qinghao (*Artemisia annua* Linn) were identified for further research. These herbs were subjected to modern drug development processes, which include the extraction of active components, laboratory safety tasting, and clinical research (Fig. 6.4).

Question and Answer

7. How to identify the TCM candidate? [Multiple-choice question]

A. Investigating folk prescriptions to compile a list of herbal medicine
B. Conducting preclinical studies to screen effective and low-toxicant herbal medicine
C. Investigating resource of the herbal medicine
D. Others, please explain______

Reference answer:

– Open question.

All the steps are necessary, but more need to be done. Please refer to FDA's website for more information on drug development process.

https://www.fda.gov/patients/learn-about-drug-and-device-approvals/drug-development-process

Recommended discussion time:

– 6 min

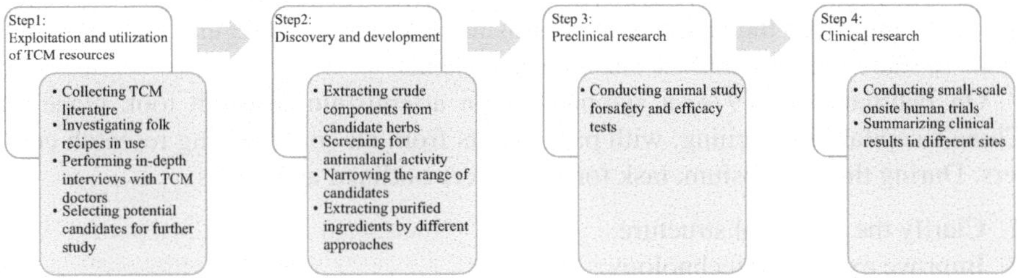

Fig. 6.4 China's drug development flow—Traditional Chinese Medicine Group (Liu et al. 2022; Tu et al. 2015)

6.3 Part 3. What Did We Learn?

6.3.1 *Information 6*

The results of artemisinin clinical trials.

From 1973 to 1978, clinical trials of artemisinin involved 2099 malaria patients from across the country, including chloroquine-resistant cases and cerebral malaria cases. The outcomes were promising, with almost all cases showing positive responses. Ten fatalities occurred due to unrelated complications during the trial.

Artemisinin: from discovery to worldwide acknowledgment (Liu et al. 2022).

In 1976, it was discovered that a plant chemist in Yugoslavia was independently isolating and extracting natural compounds from local *Artemisia annua* Linn. Upon confirming that these compounds were identical to artemisinin, Chinese researchers decided to publish their findings in journals to unveil the chemical structure of artemisinin (Note: The national patent system was established after 1985).

In 1977, the first paper on artemisinin, titled "Artemisinin: A New Type of Sesquiterpene Lactone," was published in the third issue of Scientific Bulletin. This publication disclosed the structural formula of artemisinin without explicitly mentioning its antimalarial efficacy. The second paper, titled "The structure and reaction of artemisinin," was published in *Acta chemica Sinica*, Vol. 37, No. 2, in 1979. In November 1979, the third paper, titled "The crystal structure and absolute configuration of artemisinin," was published in *Science of China*, Vol B, No. 11. An English version of this paper was later introduced in *Scientia Sinica*, Vol. 23, No. 3, 1980. Then, in 1979, a paper titled "The Research on the Antimalarial Drug Artemisinin," was published in the Pharmaceutical Bulletin No. 2 (14 (49–53) (now renamed as the *Journal of Chinese Medicine*). This review extensively covered artemisinin's efficacy, toxicology, pharmacodynamics, and clinical trials involving artemisinin tablets, oil solution, oil suspension agent and water suspension agent. The English version of this article was published in the twelfth issue of *Chinese Medical Journal* on page 811–816 in 1979. In 1980, the report "Research on Artemisinin Derivatives" was published in the fourth issue of the Pharmaceutical Sciences Bulletin, reporting the clinical effects of 804-sodium (artesunate) in 186 cases.

Question and Answer

11. What do you think are the reasonable procedures for developing new traditional medicine? Is the procedure for developing Artemisinin consistent with your country's? [Choose the correct answers and put them in the right order]

A. Collecting TM material(prescriptions and herbal medicine samples)
B. Conducting clinical trial observation
C. Carrying out pharmacological toxicity study
D. Extracting effective ingredients

E. Conducting structure determination
F. Putting it into market
G. Applying for a patent
H. Publishing results in the scientific community
I. Getting government approval
J. Obtaining permission from international organizations
K. Conducting study on dosage forms

Reference answer:

- China's R&D on artemisinin: IADCKBEH.
- Ideal R&D pattern on traditional medicine: ACDKBEGJHF.

Recommended discussion time:

- 12 min

Question and Answer

12. What are the key elements of a successful government-led drug R&D according to the artemisinin discovery history? Which step is the hardest to accomplish in your country?

(Hint: Government commitment; resource; funding…)

Reference answer:

- Open question.

Recommended discussion time:

- 9 min

Question and Answer

13. What are some drawbacks in the modern perspective of Artemisinin R&D?

Reference answer:

- Until the issuance of China's Drug Administration Law in 1985, formal processes and records for new drug administration and approval were absent. Clinical trials lacked scientific rigor, and from 1949 to 1978, there was no protection of pharmaceutical intellectual property rights in China. This led to easy and unauthorized copying of self-developed drugs. Nowadays most patents of artemisinin-based medicines are registered by foreign pharmaceutical companies, posing a significant obstacle to further innovation in China.

- It is noteworthy that the World Health Organization's Regulation and Prequalification Department classifies regulatory agencies into stringent and those of low- and middle-income countries (LMIC). LMIC regulatory agencies often lack comprehensive standards for new drug approval. The WHO provides clear guidance to these agencies, ensuring adherence to global standards. Conducting traditional medicine R&D under WHO guidance aligns with current new drug development standards, facilitating recognition in the global market. Without such guidance, gaining international acceptance is challenging.

  Recommended discussion time:
- 9 min

Question and Answer
14. What traditional medicine could be developed in your country? Please elaborate on your reasons. [Open question]
  Recommended discussion time:
- 6 min.

Acknowledgments This work was supported by the Bill & Melinda Gates Foundation (No. INV-018913).

References

"523" (2015) The secret mission to Vietnam that spawned artemisinin. Friends Farmers (12):36
Croft AM (2007) A lesson learnt: the rise and fall of Lariam and Halfan. J R Soc Med 100(4):170–174
D'Alessandro U, Buttiëns H (2001) History and importance of antimalarial drug resistance. Trop Med Int Health 6(11):845–848
Farooq U, Mahajan RC (2004) Drug resistance in malaria. J Vector Borne Dis 41(3–4):45–53
Harrison M, Yim SV (2017) War on two fronts: the fight against parasites in Korea and Vietnam. Med Hist 61(3):401–423
Hay SI, Guerra CA, Tatem AJ, Noor AM, Snow RW (2004) The global distribution and population at risk of malaria: past, present, and future. Lancet Infect Dis 4(6):327–336
Li R, Rao Y, Zhang D (2017) The prelude to the introduction of artemisinin medicines to the world. Sci Cult Rev 14(02):50–68
Liu G, Xie Y, Sun Y, Zhang K, Ma J, Huang Y (2022) Drug research and development opportunities in low- and middle-income countries: accelerating traditional medicine through systematic utilization and comprehensive synergy. Infect Dis Poverty 11(1):27
Our World in Data. https://ourworldindata.org/. Accessed 10 Jan 2021
State Statistics Bureau. data.stats.gov.cn

Tse EG, Korsik M, Todd MH (2019) The past, present and future of anti-malarial medicines. Malar J 18(1):93
Tu Y et al (2015) Oral presentation. Interviews on the "523" Mission and Artemisinin Research and Development. Hunan Education Press, Changsha
Wernsdorfer WH, Kouznetsov RL (1980) Drug-resistant malaria—occurrence, control, and surveillance. Bull World Health Organ 58(3):341–352
Zhang J (2015) Late report: chronicles of the five-two-three project and artemisinin research and development. Yangcheng Evening News Press, Guangzhou

Chapter 7
International Promotion of Artemisinin-Based Combination Therapies

Yang-Mu Huang, Yi-Nuo Sun, Guang-Qi, LiuYu-Ming Liu, and Yan Xie

Theme
International promotion of artemisinin-based combination therapies (ACTs).

Target Audience
Policy-makers.

Learning Objectives
After completing this case study, the participant should be able to:

1. Identify key concepts for international promotion of new drugs: GLP, GMP, GCP, PQ (prequalification), NDA (new drug application).
2. Discuss the process and key stages of international promotion of new drugs.
3. List international partners and cooperation models to promote a drug globally.
4. Analyze the challenges and solutions in the international promotion of new drugs.

7.1 Background

7.1.1 The Beginning of Artemisinin Internationalization

7.1.1.1 The Start of International Collaboration

The English paper "Antimalarial Studies on Qinghaosu," initially published in the *Chinese Medicine Journal* in 1979, sparked global interest in this innovative medication. In 1980, the Scientific Working Group on the Chemotherapy of Malaria (SWG-CHEMAL) convened to discuss artemisinin and its derivatives, facilitated by

Y.-M. Huang (✉) · Y.-N. Sun · G.-Q. Liu · Y.-M. Liu·Y. Xie
Department of Global Health, Peking University School of Public Health, Beijing, People's Republic of China

Institute for Global Health, Peking University, Beijing, People's Republic of China
e-mail: ymhuang@bjmu.edu.cn

X.-N. Zhou, J.-H. Yin (eds.), *Malaria Control and Elimination in China*,
https://doi.org/10.1007/978-981-97-8719-7_7

Dr. Mahler and Mr. Qian Xinzhong of the Chinese Ministry of Public Health. This meeting underscored the significance of exploring and researching artemisinin and its derivatives in China and marked the beginning of international collaboration on artemisinin (China Cooperative Research Group 1982). Recognizing the pressing need for new antimalarial drugs, the Ministry of Public Health of China initiated a 6-year partnership with the World Health Organization (WHO). The goal of this collaboration is to evaluate these drugs and explore ways for SWG-CHEMAL to support Chinese authorities in further advancing this compound.

7.1.1.2 Advancements in Candidate Drugs Research

The fourth meeting of the SWG-CHEMAL, convened by the World Bank, United Nations Development Program, and Tropical Diseases Research (TDR), took place in Beijing from October 6–10, 1981. The meeting centered on the theme "Research on the antimalarial drug artemisinin and its derivatives." Prof. Peters' CHEMAL team launched collaborative research aimed at identifying knowledge gaps and formulating a research plan with China to explore the potential applications of dihydroartemisinin, artemether, and artesunate, which were discovered by Chinese scientists (Li et al. 2017). A number of derivatives underwent investigation for global promotion, with a particular focus on arteether, a sister drug of artesunate.

7.1.2 International Collaboration in the 1980s

7.1.2.1 Cooperation with WHO

Based on the principles outlined during the conference in October 1981, China formulated a research plan for 1982–1983. A key priority was the completion of preclinical pharmacology and toxicology testing of candidate drug preparations in accordance with international new drug registration standards. China received technical and financial assistance from WHO. In addition, the US Food and Drug Administration (FDA) received funding from WHO to facilitate Good Manufacturing Practice (GMP) inspection in China (Dana 2012).

7.1.2.2 Result of the GMP Inspection

The FDA inspection, conducted between September 18, 1982, and October 2, 1982, found that the drug's synthesis and formulation failed to meet global GMP guidelines. In response to these findings, CHEMAL proposed two potential courses of action: (1) constructing a new, GMP-compliant workshop in China or refurbishing an existing one and (2) obtaining a batch of artesunate from a non-Chinese research institute that adheres to GMP regulations (Dana 2012). The U.S. Walter Reed Army

Institute of Research (WRAIR) was recommended by WHO as a suitable research institute outside China.

7.1.2.3 Cooperation with the United States

From 1983 to 1985, China and WRAIR engaged in collaborative research and development on artesunate under the auspices of WHO. China supplied artesunate, which underwent examination in WRAIR's standard laboratory. However, until the international registration of artesunate was achieved, the scope of cooperation between the two parties was restricted to the preparation, processing of the drug, and the requisite test data. Despite this collaboration, meaningful discussions were lacking during the 2-year negotiation period, and substantial disagreements arose between the parties regarding the objectives, methods, and feasibility of implementing cooperation agreements. Concurrently, following the publication of results on artemisinin and its derivatives in China, various initiatives such as the introduction and cultivation of *Artemisia annua*, breeding and planting experiments, pharmacological research, and derivatives research abroad were fully underway.

7.1.2.4 The Failure of Cooperation and the Ignorance of Intellectual Property

In 1985, the United States military discovered *Artemisia annua*, from which they extracted artemisinin. This discovery led to the publication of an article in Science, confirming the efficacy of artemisinin. Consequently, TDR discontinued its collaborative research and development program on artesunate instability with China, shifting its focus to partnering with the United States to develop artemether. However, this multiyear collaboration ultimately proved futile. Meanwhile, foreign research on medications containing artemisinin advanced rapidly. Due to various internal issues and a lack of understanding of international drug policy, China missed the global opportunity to patent artemisinin derivatives, despite the prior knowledge of the discovery of artemisinin and its compounds.

7.1.3 Moving to a Global Stage

7.1.3.1 Foreign Cooperation

China continued its development efforts with artesunate (Zamiska and McKay 2007). Reports indicate that Kunming initially offered it for sale as a monotherapy in the late 1980s (Zamiska and McKay 2007).

The subsequent phase of development involved blending Qinghaosu with other medications that had demonstrated efficacy during initial trials in China. In the early

1990s, Chinese scientists synthesized lumefantrin, also known as benflumetol, and combined it with artemether.

CibaGeigy, later renamed Novartis (Liu et al. 2020), acquired the marketing rights for the combination outside of China and branded it as Coartem®. In 1994, Novartis entered into an agreement for further development work with a Chinese consortium. The combination underweights its initial international registration process in 1995, and in 1999, it received registration in Switzerland (Olliaro and Taylor 2003). Additional preclinical and clinical research was conducted to ensure compliance with Western drug regulations. The combination was later named Riamet® (Taylor et al. 2003) and was approved for sale in April 2009 by the FDA.

7.1.3.2 Development of ACT

The term "artemisinin [-based] combination therapy" likely emerged in the late 1980s and early 1990s, coinciding with the preliminary research conducted by François Nosten and Nicholas White in Thailand (Eastman and Fidock 2009). In June 1998, the WHO convened an informal consultation in Geneva, during which combination therapies involving artemisinin and its derivatives were first discussed and recommended for the treatment of uncomplicated malaria on a global scale. Under the supervision of WHO/TDR and with funding from the US Agency for International Development and the Wellcome Trust, innovative trials testing different combinations of ACT were carried out in nine African countries, as well as in Thailand and Peru, in the late 1990s.

By 2004, experts regarded artemisinins as the only first-line antimalarial drugs suitable for widespread use that remained effective against all chloroquine-resistant malaria parasites. Post 2004, there was a notable surge in demand for ACTs, a trend anticipated to persist (Li et al. 2017; Huang et al. 2018).

7.1.3.3 Seizing the Opportunity: The WHO Prequalification Program

Despite developments of artemisinin and its derivatives between the 1980s and 1990s, Chinese pharmaceutical companies faced challenges in accessing foreign markets due to stringent quality requirements imposed by importing nations through bilateral mechanisms. In 2001, WHO launched the Prequalification Program (WHO-PQ) for drugs, diagnostic reagents, vaccines, and other fields for anti-AIDS, antimalarial, and antituberculosis drugs. This initiative mandated that pharmaceutical companies producing antimalarial drugs must obtain WHO-PQ certification to be listed in the WHO procurement catalog (Ma et al. 2020). Under this program, international funds or nongovernmental organizations can procure products meeting PQ certification standards and distribute them in underdeveloped nations and regions, notably in Africa. Drug prequalification can be achieved in two ways:

expedited approval via stringent regulatory authority (SRA), or comprehensive review encompassing certification of GMP, good laboratory practice (GLP), good clinical practice (GCP), and other standards aligned with international norms (e.g., FDA). Guilin Pharmaceutical Co., Ltd.'s artesunate became the first Chinese product to attain WHO-PQ certification in 2005 (Eastman and Fidock 2009).

7.2 Part 1. Determining the Drug and Timing for International Promotion

7.2.1 Background

Following the discovery of artemisinin and its three derivatives (dihydroartemisinin, artemether, and artesunate) by Chinese artists, efforts were made to make these medications globally available. In the 1980s, China sought assistance from WHO and collaboratively convened a meeting to establish research agenda and explore potential applications of artemisinin and its derivatives in malaria prevention initiatives. During the conference, China and WHO prioritized the development of water-soluble artesunate for treating cerebral malaria, with a preference for using artemisinin or its derivatives outside of China. However, subsequent collaborations were not successful, and concerns about the instability of artesunate led to its development being halted. In 1985, attention shifted to its sister drug, arteether, developed by the United States, which ultimately proved to be an unsuccessful choice.

Question and Answer

1. Name possible drugs in your country and analyze whether they meet the requirements and conditions for international promotion. Elaborate from the perspective of global demand, drug advantages, internal supportive environment, urgency of needs, national interest, and global welfare.

Reference answer:

- Global burden of malaria.
- The efficacy, adverse reactions, pharmacology, price, course of treatment, medication adherence, drug resistance of the medicine and competitive medicines.
- The urgency of need for new drugs.
- National interest and global welfare.

7.3 Part 2. The Process and Key Considerations for International Promotion

7.3.1 Background

The international promotion of new drugs involves fulfilling admission qualifications set by target countries and adhering to quality management standard certifications for various stages of drug research, production, and clinical trials in each country. In collaboration with WHO, efforts have been made in China to facilitate this process. This includes supporting the FDA in conducting GMP inspections and providing WHO with GLP and GMP procedural documents to expedite entry of new drugs into the international market. However, challenges persist, as clinical trials were restricted in China due to the absence of GMP inspection approval. In response, WHO has recommended collaborating with an accredited organization outside of China to address the GMP compliance issue.

Question and Answer

2. What are the main international drug practices involved in the process of international promotion of new drugs? (select all that apply)

A. Good manufacture practice, GMP
B. Good laboratory practice, GLP
C. Good clinical practice, GCP
D. Good supplying practice, GSP
E. Others

Reference answer: ABCDE

- In the process of international promotion of new drugs, it is necessary to obtain the admittance qualification of target countries, with each country implementing a quality management standard certification system for drug research, production, clinical trials, and other related activities. The main standards include the following:
- GMP is a set of mandatory standards applicable to pharmaceutical, food, and other industries. It requires enterprises to adhere to hygienic quality requirements concerning raw materials, personnel, facilities and equipment, production process, packaging and transportation, and quality control. It establishes operational guidelines to enhance the hygienic environment, identify production process issues, and institute improvements.
- GLP is the basic principle for preclinical drug research. It includes various aspects such as experimental design, operation, record-keeping, reporting, and supervision of drug safety evaluation in nonclinical drug research settings. GLP serves as a fundamental measure to improve the quality of new drug research from its inception and ensure public safety.

- GCP sets the standard for the entire clinical trial process, covering scheme design, organization, implementation, inspection, examination, record-keeping, analysis and summary, and reporting. It is formulated by various countries' regulatory bodies as a standardization requirement for conducting new drug clinical trials. Compliance with GCP ensures high-quality clinical research and safeguards the rights and interests of trial participants.
- GSP is a set of management procedures aimed at controlling all factors that could lead to quality incidents in the circulation of pharmaceutical products. GSP is designed to prevent quality incidents and ensure the quality of pharmaceutical products throughout their production, distribution, and sales processes. It serves as a unified quality management standard for pharmaceutical enterprises.
- Additionally, there are other standard such as good agricultural practice (GAP), and good extraction practice (cGEP), which are specifically applicable to TCM.

Question and Answer

3. What are the difficulties of international promotion for developing countries? (select all that apply)

A. International promotion process requires significant financial resources
B. International promotion process involves lengthy timelines (especially for clinical trials)
C. Technical facilities in developing countries need improvements
D. There is a significant gap between the drug management standards of developing countries and developed countries (such as GMP)
E. Protecting the rights and interests of developing countries is challenging

Reference answer:ABCDE

7.3.2 Background

In 1987, Guilin Pharmaceutical Co., Ltd. developed artesunate and obtained the National Number 001 New Drug Certificate. Nevertheless, there were still significant obstacles to overcome before artemisinin medications could be sold internationally. These included the stringent drug quality requirements set by the importing nations under bilateral mechanisms, as well as the expensive and time-consuming nature of the procedure.

The introduction of WHO-PQ certification marked a change. Achieving this certification enables companies to pass national standard certifications, potentially waiving the need for inspections by drug importing countries. This opened doors for Chinese pharmaceutical companies to access the global markets, including Europe, America, Japan, and other developed regions. However, discrepancies persist between international standards and relevant quality standards in China. Entering the WHO procurement catalog requires substantial financial resources and international management experiences, posing challenges for Chinese businesses.

Despite these challenges, Guilin Pharmaceutical Co., Ltd. has remained committed to independent research and development. As the first to achieve prequalification for artemisinin-based in China, it paved the way for further international market expansion and promotion of artesunate in malaria-endemic regions like Africa. As of 2021, the companies have successfully prequalified 21 of its antimalarial products (see Table 7.1 below).

Question and Answer

4. What are the benefits that pharmaceutical enterprises gain after passing WHO-PQ? (short answer question)

Reference answer:

1. Overcoming technical barriers. WHO-PQ certification provides a high-level "pass permit," allowing entry into the international pharmaceutical market, overcoming technical barriers in developed countries, obtaining GMP certification meeting international requirements, and avoiding inspections by other importing countries.
2. Expanding international business. WHO-PQ certification significantly reduces the difficulty of international export business and enables access to global high-end markets, such as Europe, America, Japan, and other developed countries or regions.
3. Enhancing international recognition and promoting future cooperation. WHO-PQ certification facilitate inclusion of drugs on the WHO procurement list, recognized by many international organizations and institutions such as TGF (global fund), MMV (malaria drug risk fund), UNICEF (United Nations Children's fund), gates foundation (Bill and Melinda Gates Foundation), MSF (Doctors without Borders) and nongovernmental public welfare organizations. This enhances enterprise visibility and lays the groundwork for future collaborations.

Table 7.1 21 Guilin Pharmaceutical Co., Ltd.'s antimalarial medicines that passed WHO-PQ

Applicant	International nonproprietary name (INN)	Dosage form and strength	Date of prequalification
Guilin Pharmaceutical Co Ltd—China	Artesunate	Tablet 50 mg	21-Dec-05
	Amodiaquine (hydrochloride)	Tablet, film-coated 150 mg	30-Aug-07
	Amodiaquine (hydrochloride) + artesunate	Amodiaquine (hydrochloride) tablet + artesunate tablet 150 mg + 50 mg	30-Aug-07
	Artesunate + sodium bicarbonate + sodium chloride	– (Vial + ampoule); 60 mg/vial +50 mg/mL + 45 mg/5 mL	5-Nov-10
	Pyrimethamine/sulfadoxine + artesunate	Pyrimethamine/sulfadoxine tablet + artesunate tablet 25 mg/500 mg + 50 mg	24-May-12
	Pyrimethamine/sulfadoxine + artesunate	Tablets + tablets 25 mg/500 mg + 100 mg	18-Dec-18
	Amodiaquine (hydrochloride)/artesunate	Tablet 67.5 mg/25 mg	16-Nov-12
	Amodiaquine (hydrochloride)/artesunate	Tablet 135 mg/50 mg	16-Nov-12
	Amodiaquine (hydrochloride)/artesunate	Tablet 270 mg/100 mg	16-Nov-12
	Artesunate + sodium bicarbonate + sodium chloride	Artesunate powder for injection + sodium bicarbonate solvent solution for injection + sodium chloride solvent solution for injection 30 mg/vial +5% m/v + 0.9% m/v	23-May-13
	Artesunate + sodium bicarbonate + sodium chloride	Artesunate powder for injection + sodium bicarbonate solvent solution for injection + sodium chloride solvent solution for injection 120 mg/vial +5% m/v + 0.9% m/v	23-May-13
	Pyrimethamine/sulfadoxine + amodiaquine (hydrochloride)	Pyrimethamine/sulfadoxine tablets + amodiaquine (hydrochloride) film-coated tablets 25 mg/500 mg + 150 mg	20-Oct-14
	Pyrimethamine/sulfadoxine	Tablet 25 mg/500 mg	31-Oct-18
	Pyrimethamine/sulfadoxine + amodiaquine (hydrochloride)	Pyrimethamine/sulfadoxine + amodiaquine (hydrochloride) dispersible tablets 12.5 mg/250 mg + 76.5 mg	21-Aug-18

Applicant	International nonproprietary name (INN)	Dosage form and strength	Date of prequalification
	Pyrimethamine/sulfadoxine + amodiaquine (hydrochloride)	Pyrimethamine/sulfadoxine + amodiaquine (hydrochloride) dispersible tablets 25 mg/500 mg + 153 mg	21-Aug-18
	Dihydroartemisinin/ piperaquine (phosphate)	Tablet, film-coated 40 mg/320 mg	19-Nov-19
	Dihydroartemisinin/ piperaquine (phosphate)	Tablet, dispersible 40 mg/320 mg	19-Nov-19
	Dihydroartemisinin/ piperaquine (phosphate)	Tablet, film-coated 80 mg/640 mg	19-Nov-19
	Dihydroartemisinin/ piperaquine (phosphate)	Tablet, dispersible 20 mg/160 mg	19-Nov-19
	Dihydroartemisinin/ piperaquine (phosphate)	Tablet, film-coated 60 mg/480 mg	16-Sep-20
	Dihydroartemisinin/ piperaquine (phosphate)	Tablet, dispersible 30 mg/240 mg	25-Nov-20

Question and Answer

5. What are the challenges for developing countries to pass WHO-PQ? (short answer question)

Reference answer:

1. Technical barriers: WHO-PQ certification strictly supervises equipment, environment, and quality, adhering to international standards.
2. Financial barrier: Obtaining WHO-PQ certification is time-consuming and requires substantial financial investments.
3. International competition: Developing countries face competition from pharmaceutical companies in Europe and America.
4. Information channel barriers: Developing countries often lack experience in international affairs, leading to challenges such as delayed information reception, ineffective communication, and language barriers in international certification processes.

Question and Answer

6. What factors do you think contributed to the success of Guilin Pharma in passing the WHO-PQ? (short answer question)

Reference answer:

1. Internal factors

Enterprise initiatives: Guilin pharmaceutical Corp demonstrated proactive enterprise initiatives by continuously innovating, seizing opportunities, and strategically pursuing international development goals. It aimed to penetrate markets in African countries with high disease burden, timing their entries into the WHO procurement catalogue and applying for WHO-PQ certification strategically.

2. External factors

(a) External cooperation

It made rational use of external resources, by establishing liaison mechanisms with regulatory agencies and relevant governmental bodies to update technical guidelines, train personnel, and seek technical support. Collaboration with contract research organizations helped the company overcome quality standards and technical barriers.

(b) Policy support

Initiatives like WHO's recommendation of artemisinins for malaria treatment since 2001, along with goals set by international organizations like the African union to "eliminating malaria by 2030," provided crucial policy backing for China's artemisinin drugs to enter the African market and obtain WHO-PQ certification.

Question and Answer

7. What is the significance of Guilin pharmaceutical co., ltd.'s series of drugs passing WHO-PQ from different perspectives?

Reference answer:

Its significance can be analyzed from the perspectives of pharmaceutical enterprises, countries, and the international community. This analysis can be combined with the internationalization of drugs to promote their roles as public goods and contribute to the realization of a global community of human destiny.

7.4 Part 3. External Participants and Approaches to Collaborative International Drug Promotion

7.4.1 Background

In 1979, global interest in a new medication was sparked by the publication of an English paper titled "Antimalarial Studies on Qinghaosu," in the *Chinese Medicine Journal*. This prompted China and the WHO to initiate a 6-year collaboration in 1980 to promote artemisinin internationally. Due to China's technological and equipment limitations, WHO provided assistance in 1983 by facilitating collaboration with the United States. Despite receiving financial, technical, and other support from the WHO, this cooperation ultimately failed.

Question and Answer

8. How can external cooperation and support be sought for challenges that cannot be addressed domestically? (short answer question)

Reference answer:

1. Forms of cooperation

Multilateral mechanism: Establish multilateral cooperation with global and local international organizations and countries to promote international promotion.

Bilateral mechanism: Engage in one-to-one cooperation with developed countries or other nations possessing higher technical and economic capabilities.

2. Fields of cooperation

Funds: Seek financial support from international organizations and developed countries to address funding requirements involved in international drug promotion.

Technology: Solicit technical support from international organizations and developed countries to facilitate technical cooperation. This may involve initiatives such introducing technical facilities, providing training for technical personnel, addressing issues related to drug production management standards (GMP), and advancing clinical trials.

Question and Answer

9. How can public-private partnerships (PPPs) be promoted in the process of promoting new drugs? (short answer question)

Reference answer:

PPPs refers to cooperative arrangements between the public and private sectors aimed at providing public projects or services traditionally overseen by the public sector. The public generally refers to the government, public organizations, institutions, while the private sector mainly comprises pharmaceutical companies.

Public sector:

- Standardizing the pharmaceutical market and formulating policies can aim in advancing pharmaceutical research and development, production, and distribution.
- Selecting the appropriate private partner based on economic strength and scientific capabilities is essential.
- Enacting robust laws to ensure effective functioning of PPPs.

Private sector:

- Leveraging its expertise, the private sector can lead industry operations, utilizing its strengths in fundraising and management.
- Contributing technology and knowledge to collaborative efforts is crucial for the private sector's involvement.

Both sectors:

- Clear division of labor, mutual trust, shared responsibility, and risk are vital for successful partnerships.

Question and Answer
10. Summarize the cooperation and financing models used in promoting artemisinin, and propose potential cooperation and financing models applicable to your country. (short answer question)
Reference answer: (open question)

- Cooperation model:
  Bilateral mechanism: China initially collaborated with WHO but encountered GMP and other technical problems.
  Multilateral mechanism: The US later joined the cooperation, forming a multilateral mechanism through WHO coordination to collectively address technical challenges.
- Financing model:
  Primarily through WHO and international foundations, such as the World Bank, Clinton Foundation, and Bill & Melinda Gates Foundation.

Question and Answer
11. What are the advantages and disadvantages of international cooperation in international promotion? (short answer question)
Reference answer:
Advantages:

- Compensating for technical gaps.
- Access to financial assistance.
- Standardization alignment.
- Accelerating clinical trials.
- Enhancing international recognition.

Disadvantages:

- Risk to R&D country interests.
- Potential delays due to disagreements.

Subsequently, WHO discontinued its collaborative research and development project on artesunate stability with China, opting instead to focus on partnering with the United States to develop artemether. During the two and a half years of "space separation cooperation" between China and the United States from 1983 to 1985, meaningful discussions did not materialize. Significant disparities existed between the parties concerning the goals, implementation, and feasibility of the cooperation arrangement, leading to an unsuccessful collaboration in the end.

7.4.2 Background

Foreign research on artemisinin-containing medications surged during the years of collaboration between China, the United States, and WHO. However, due to internal challenges and a lack of familiarity with international drug policies, China missed the opportunity to patent artemisinin derivatives globally, despite prior knowledge of their discovery. Nevertheless, Chinese scientists developed an artemether-lumefantrine combination in the early 1990s. Novartis, formerly Ciba Geigy, acquired rights to market the combination outside of China under the Coartem® name, agreeing to pay royalties and a significant sum upfront. The Academy of Military Medical Science in China purportedly owned the intellectual property rights, which Novartis co-owned or leased until 2011. Following studies for international registration initiated in 1995, and the combination was registered in Switzerland in 1999. Additional preclinical and clinical research ensured compliance with Western drug regulations. Marketed as Riamet®, it gained FDA approval in 2009. Additionally, in the 1980s, China provided WHO with a kilogram of purified artemisinin for testing, potentially leading to intellectual property concerns.

Question and Answer

12. How can the rights and interests of R&D countries be protected in international promotion? (short answer question)

Reference answer:

- Applying for patents is essential to protect intellectual property rights in the field of medicine, including all intellectual achievements related to medical industry inventions and creations. Drug patents play a crucial role in the development process due to its high difficulty, investment, risk, and duration. Therefore, patent protection is sought during both the development and research stages of new drugs.
- Drug patents typically offer a protection period of 20 years in countries like China, the United States, and Japan. They not only empower R&D endeavors but also serve as institutional safeguards and foundational assets for subsequent drug-related patent technology R&D. This, in turn, fosters healthy and robust growths in the pharmaceutical industry.

- Internationally, the world property organization (WIPO) established the patent cooperation treaty (PCT) on June 19, 1970. The PCT enables applicants to submit a single "international" patent application, valid across all member countries simultaneously. This treaty facilitates international patent protection and streamlines the global patent application process.

7.5 Part 4. Strategies and Challenges for Local Drug Promotion

7.5.1 Background

Launching a new medication in the global market involves several crucial steps. Initial processes include WHO prequalification, national registration, and local market authorization. However, beyond these steps lies the key to success, exemplified by a Chinese pharmaceutical company's triumph with its artemisinin series products in international markets. This success is attributed to the company's adept foreign marketing strategies.

Through extensive and long-term research conducted across various African countries, the company allocated resources to its most competitive products, particularly targeting the artemisinin injection market. This market segment, within the fiercely competitive African antimalarial drug market, sees significant contention among numerous international pharmaceutical groups and Indian generic drug manufacturers. Currently, the company's artemisinin injection holds a remarkable market share of over 90%.

Critical to executing their localization strategy, the company built offices and wholly owned subsidiaries in African nations, as well as forming dedicated teams to manage drug sales and clinical promotions on the ground. Furthermore, the company actively engaged with governments and international organizations from exporting nations to participate in public welfare. These efforts included providing free medical care and drug donations, all while building a strong brand reputation.

Question and Answer
13. Please reflect on methods to enhance the adoption of the designated application area and the rationale behind selecting products from your country. (short answer question)

Reference answer:

- High disease burden in the region.
- Significant treatment effect.
- High drug safety.
- Competitive pricing.
- Ease of medication administration.

Question and Answer

14. Given the varying populations' suitability for drugs, what preparations do you believe are necessary? (short answer question)

Reference answer:

- Local phase III clinical trials.
  Phase III clinical trial is the confirmation stage for therapeutic efficacy. These trials aim to further verify the drug's effectiveness and safety in patients with targeted indications, evaluate the balance between benefits and risks, and provide sufficient basis for drug registration review. Conducting local clinical trials allows for the verification of the drug's efficacy and safety across diverse local populations, thereby assessing its applicability and providing a foundation for its local promotion.
- Post-market surveillance.
  Post-market surveillance involves ongoing monitoring of adverse reactions, offering a scientific basis for drug safety reassessment. Continuous safety monitoring of drug post-market is important. It entails investigating the drug's application in real-world clinical settings, tracking its safety and effectiveness over time, and addressing any limitations in pre-market clinical research.

Question and Answer

15. How can the issue of inconsistent usage of promoted drugs by medical personnel, resulting in diminished treatment outcomes and reputation, be effectively addressed? (short answer question)

Reference answer: (open question)

- Implement strict management protocols for drug use.
- Strengthen training and assessment procedures for medical personnel.
- Improve posttreatment monitoring and patient follow-up evaluations.

Acknowledgments This work was supported by the Bill & Melinda Gates Foundation (No. INV-018913).

References

China Cooperative Research Group (1982) China Cooperative Research Group on Qinghaosu and its derivatives as antimalarials. Chemical studies on Qinghaosu (artemisinine). J Tradit Chin Med 2(1):3–8

Dana G (2012) Dalrymple, Artemisia annua, Artemisinin, ACTs & Malaria Control in Africa: tradition, science and public policy. Politics and Prose Bookstore, Washington, DC

Eastman R, Fidock D (2009) Artemisinin-based combination therapies: a vital tool in efforts to eliminate malaria. Nat Rev Microbiol 12:864–874
Huang Y, Pan K, Peng D, Stergachis A (2018) A qualitative assessment of the challenges of WHO prequalification for anti-malarial drugs in China. Malar J 17(1):149
Li R, Rao Y, Zhang D (2017) The prelude to the introduction of artemisinin medicines to the world. Sci Cult Rev 14(02):50–68
Liu K, Zuo H, Li G, Yu H, Hu Y (2020) Global research on artemisinin and its derivatives: perspectives from patents. Pharmacol Res 159:105048
Ma N, Zhang Z, Liao F, Jiang T, Tu Y (2020) The birth of artemisinin. Pharmacol Ther 216:107658
Olliaro PL, Taylor WR (2003) Antimalarial compounds: from bench to bedside. J Exp Biol 206(Pt 21):3753–3759
Taylor WR, Rigal J, Olliaro PL (2003) Drug resistant falciparum malaria and the use of artesunate-based combinations: focus on clinical trials sponsored by TDR. J Vector Borne Dis 40(3–4):65–72
Zamiska N, McKay B (2007) Global health, China's price in malaria clash. Wall Street J:A1–A14

The manufacturer's authorised representative in the EU is Springer Nature Customer Service Centre GmbH, Europaplatz 3, 69115 Heidelberg, Germany. If you have any concerns regarding our products, please contact ProductSafety@springernature.com

Printed and bound by CPI Group (UK) Ltd, Croydon, CR0 4YY

01/10/2026

02225944-0015